Practical Workbook of

HUMAN PHYSIOLOGY

Practical Workbook of HUMAN PHYSIOLOGY

SECOND EDITION

K Sri Nageswari MD FABMS IFME
Professor
Department of Physiology
Dr VRK Women's Medical College
Hyderabad, Telangana, India

Formerly, Professor and Head
Department of Physiology
Professor In-Charge–Academics
Government Medical College
Chandigarh, India

Rajeev Sharma MD
Professor and Head
Department of Physiology
Guru Gobind Singh Medical College
Faridkot, Punjab, India

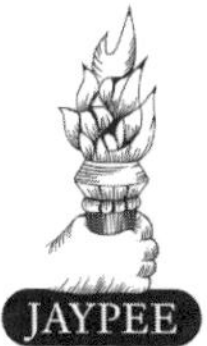

JAYPEE BROTHERS MEDICAL PUBLISHERS
The Health Sciences Publisher
New Delhi | London

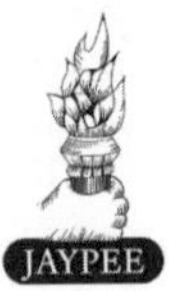

Jaypee Brothers Medical Publishers (P) Ltd

Headquarters

Jaypee Brothers Medical Publishers (P) Ltd
23/23-B, Ansari Road, Daryaganj
New Delhi 110 002, India
Phone:+91-11-23272143, +91-11-23272703
+91-11-23282021, +91-11-23245672
E-mail: jaypee@jaypeebrothers.com

Corporate Office

Jaypee Brothers Medical Publishers (P) Ltd.
4838/24, Ansari Road, Daryaganj
New Delhi 110 002, India
Phone: +91-11-43574357
Fax: +91-11-43574314
E-mail: jaypee@jaypeebrothers.com

Overseas Offices

J P Medical Ltd
83 Victoria Street, London
SW1H 0HW (UK)
Phone: +44 20 3170 8910
E-mail: info@jpmedpub.com

EU GPSR Authorised Representative
Logos Europe, 9 rue Nicolas Poussin
17000, La Rochelle, France
Phone: +33 (0) 6 67 93 73 78
E-mail: Contact@logoseurope.eu

Website: www.jaypeebrothers.com
Website: www.jaypeedigital.com

Inquiries for bulk sales may be solicited at: jaypee@jaypeebrothers.com

Practical Workbook of Human Physiology

First Edition: 2006
Second Edition: 2018

Reprint: 2024, **2025**

ISBN 978-93-5270-145-2

Printed at: Sterling Graphics Pvt. Ltd. India.

Dedicated to

My husband Dr KR Sarma
for his enormous patience, support and encouragement

My children, Sharat-Sunita, Ravi-Raji, and Aarati-Ram
for their abundant love and affection

My father Late Major VS Rao
for his everlasting discipline, moral and ethical values
and

My mother Late Mrs VVV Lakshmi
for her great dedication and commitment as a single parent

—K Sri Nageswari

My parents, my wife Ritu and
My children Tushar and Twisha

—Rajeev Sharma

PREFACE

Practical Workbook of Human Physiology has been prepared for the first year MBBS students of various medical colleges across the country; it will also benefit the students of first year BDS, BAMS, BHMS, BPT and MSc Physiology courses. Different textbooks of physiology and clinical medicine as well as relevant websites have been consulted for the preparation of the workbook.

New experiments have been added in the second edition. *Practical Manual of Haematology* authored by Dr K Sri Nageswari and Dr Anamika Kothari and published by M/s Jaypee Brothers Medical Publishers (P) Ltd is now clubbed with this workbook as a separate chapter, "Haematology Experiments". As per feedback from teachers and students, the text of some of the practicals has also been revised.

The contents describe experiments and demonstration experiments under the main headings of Respiratory System, Cardiovascular System, Central Nervous System, Reproductive System, Nerve Muscle Physiology Experiments, Mammalian Experiments and Haematology Experiments. Under the heading "Experiments", the list of experiments are given which are to be performed by the students themselves. Demonstration experiments are those where the students are given practical demonstrations of the experiments. During the Vertical Orientation Programme, the students visit various clinical departments to learn about Echocardiography, Holter and Stress ECG, latest trends and techniques adopted for testing pulmonary functions and safe blood transfusion procedures. This programme encourages the students to learn physiology and pathophysiology of various ailments through interaction with clinical departments.

The authors are of the opinion that the book will provide all the pertinent experimental and clinical material related to different experiments at one place for the benefit of the first year medical students and students of allied disciplines in the subject of physiology.

We are thankful to Dr Anjana MS and Dr Suneet Khurana, for their help in the preparation of the practical workbook. The secretarial assistance provided by Ms Satinder Kaur and Ms Parminder Kaur is duly acknowledged.

K Sri Nageswari

Rajeev Sharma

CONTENTS

PLATE 1

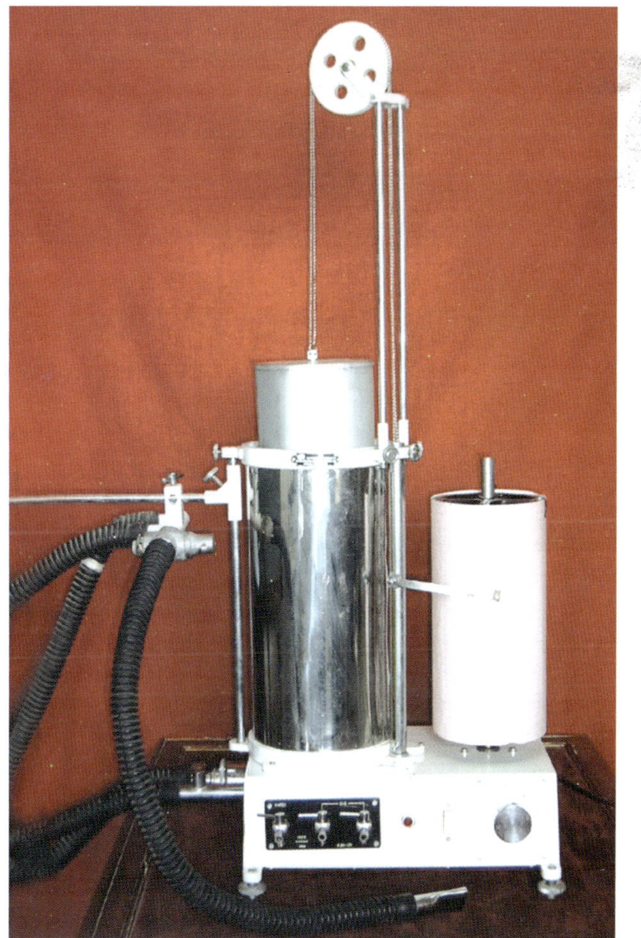

Fig. 1: Benedict Roth apparatus

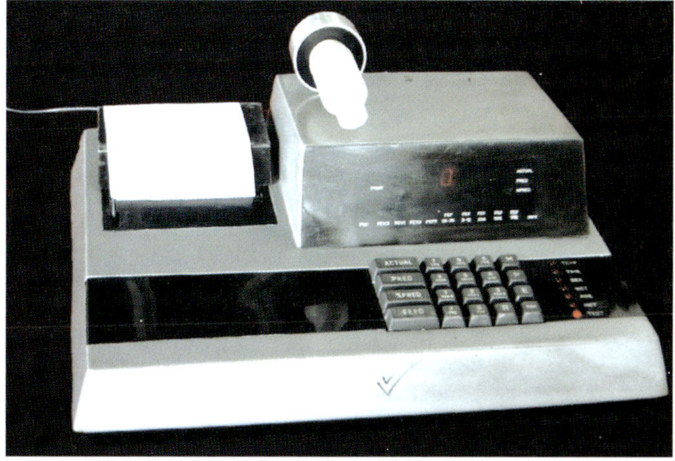

Fig. 2: Medspiror

PLATE 2

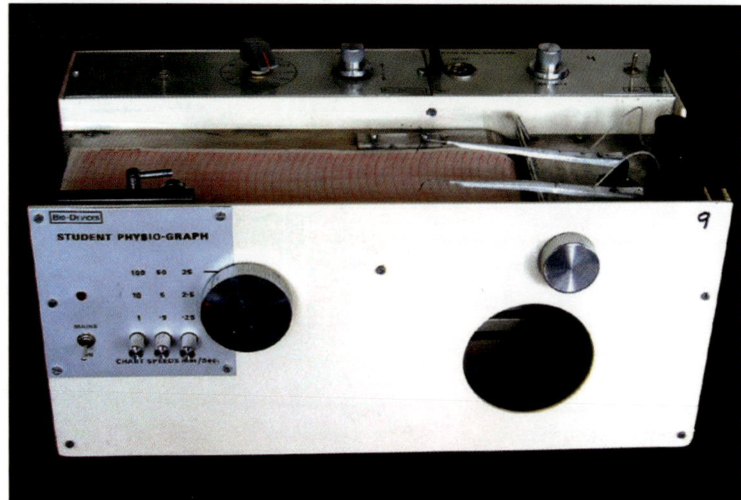

Fig. 3: Physiograph

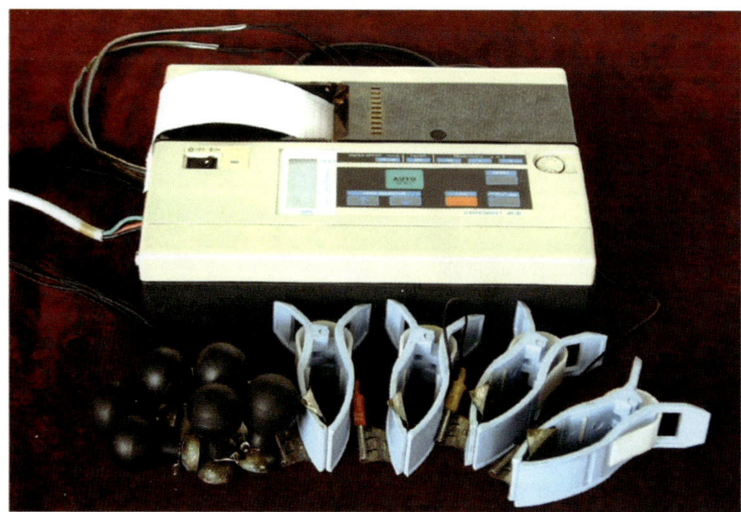

Fig. 4: Electrocardiograph

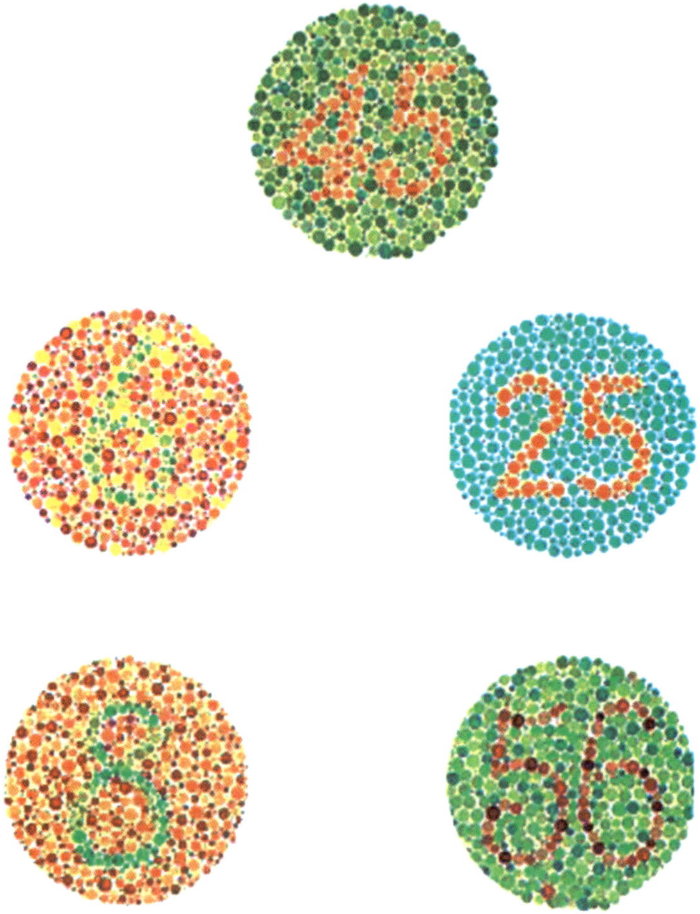

Fig. 5: Ishihara's pseudoisochromatic color plates

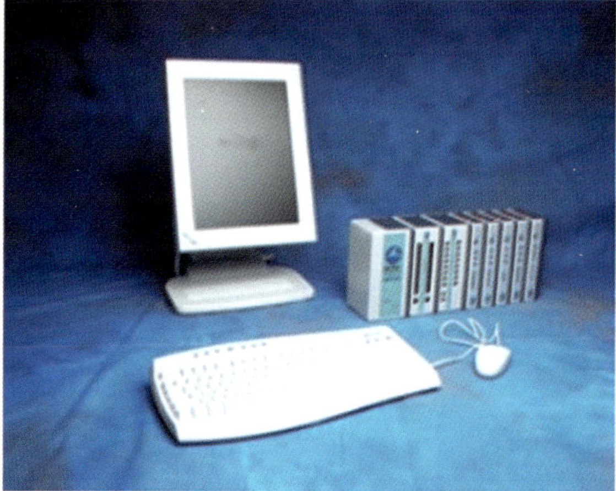

Fig. 6: 16 channel data acquisition and analysis system (Biopac)

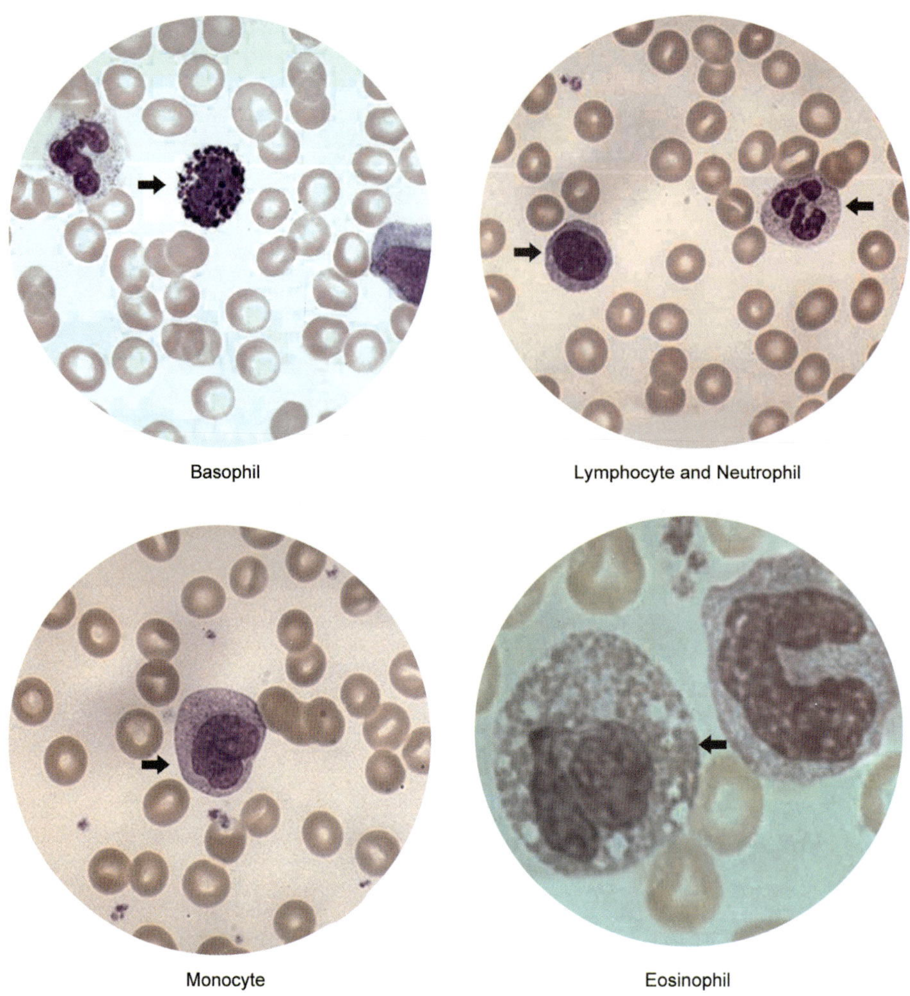

Fig. 7: Peripheral blood smear showing various cells

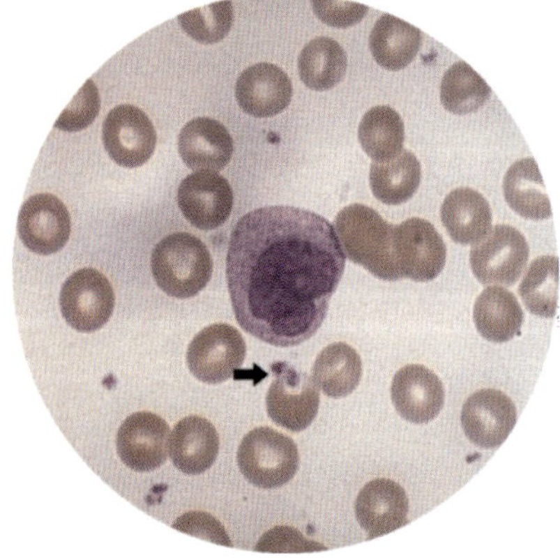

Fig. 8: Peripheral blood smear showing platelets

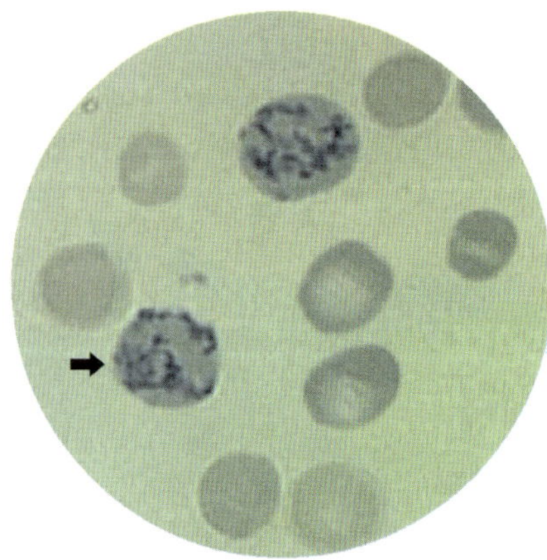

Fig. 9: Peripheral blood smear showing reticulocytes

Chapter 1

Respiratory System

EXPERIMENT NO. 1

AIM: TO EXAMINE THE RESPIRATORY SYSTEM OF THE SUBJECT

Procedure

The respiratory system of the subject should be examined with the person comfortably seated in erect position with complete exposure of chest in good light. The general physical examination should also be carried out at the same time which includes noting down the temperature, pulse, blood pressure, jugular venous pressure and looking for abnormal signs like pallor, oedema, cyanosis, clubbing and lymphadenopathy.

Respiratory examination should be carried out under four headings:

- Inspection
- Palpation
- Percussion
- Auscultation.

Inspection

The subject is asked to sit comfortably, bare-chested. The rate, rhythm, depth, expansion, type of respiration and shape of the chest is noted.

- *Rate:* Normal rate is 14–16 breaths/minute. Increased rate of respiration is called tachypnoea. Tachypnoea occurs in newborns, infants, children, females, with exercise, emotion, excitement, etc.
- *Rhythm:* Regular or irregular.
  - *Irregular rhythm:* Any abnormalities in rhythm like Cheyne-Stokes breathing or Biot's breathing are noted.
  - *Cheyne-Stokes breathing:* Alternating periods of apnoea and hyperventilation. This type of breathing is seen in left ventricular failure, brain damage, high altitude, after voluntary hyperventilation.
  - *Biot's breathing:* Irregularity in depth and rhythm with pauses in between. Seen in meningitis.
  - *Kussmaul breathing:* Increased rate and depth of respiration (air hunger). Seen in metabolic acidosis like in diabetes.

- *Depth:* Whether the breathing is shallow or deep is noted down. Shallow breathing occurs with bronchial asthma and deep breathing with brain damage or uraemia.
- *Expansion:* Should be measured with a measuring tape, whether expansion is symmetric or not. It is abnormal in emphysema, pleural effusion, pnuemothorax and fibrosis of lung.
- *Type of respiration:* It may be thoracic or abdominal or thoracoabdominal.
- *Shape of the chest:* Normal shape of the chest is bilaterally symmetrical and elliptical. Some common abnormal shapes of the chest are:
  - *Pigeon shape:* Rickets in children
  - *Barrel shape:* Anteroposterior diameter of chest increases in emphysema, bronchial asthma, fibrosis of the lung.
  - *Scoliosis:* Lateral bending of vertebral column.
  - *Kyphosis:* Forward bending of vertebral column.
  - *Kyphoscoliosis:* Common in tuberculosis of spine.

Palpation

1. Approximating the tips of the thumbs in the midline and keeping the fingertips in fixed position on lower rib cage, symmetry of expansion of the chest is assessed by noting the degree of displacement of thumbs on either side due to expansion. Normally the expansion is more than 5 cm at the base of lungs.
2. Position of the trachea is noted. The trachea is felt in the suprasternal notch, by insinuating fingers on both sides of it. Its placement in relation to the suprasternal notch is noted.
3. *Vocal fremitus:* With the ulnar border of hand placed on chest of the subject along the intercostal space, subject is asked to repetitively utter some word like ninety-nine or one-two-three. The intensity of vibrations transmitted in the corresponding area on the two sides of the chest in each intercostal space is assessed. This should be equal on both sides.
4. *Position of apex beat:* It is felt in the left 5th intercostal space, 1 cm internal to the midclavicular line.

Percussion

- Percussion of different areas of chest is done to note down the degree of resonance from the more resonant to the less resonant areas.
- The middle finger (pleximeter finger) of left hand is placed on the part to be percussed and its middle phalanx is struck with the tip of the middle finger (percussing finger) of right hand, taking care that the movement of striking hand should be at the wrist joint. Percussion note is compared on the two corresponding areas of the chest always.
- Percussion should be carried out in three to four areas on anterior chest wall, in the axilla and four areas on the back, comparing left with the right.
- The intercostal area where hepatic dullness appears is noted to demarcate the boundary of liver.
- Any additional site of dullness/tympani is noted.

Auscultation

For auscultation, the patient should be in sitting position. He should breathe deeply and regularly with the mouth open and face turned to other side.

- Breath sounds and their character

- Character of vocal resonance
- Presence of added sounds.

Breath sounds

Note whether the breath sounds are vesicular or bronchial.

- *Vesicular breath sounds:* These are produced by passage of air in and out of normal lung tissue and heard all over the chest in normal condition. Inspiratory sounds are fairly intense and heard for the duration twice that of the duration of expiration. The quality of the sounds is rustling and low pitched. There is no distinct pause between the end of inspiration and start of expiration.
- *Bronchial breath sounds:* Normally produced by passage of air through trachea, larynx and large bronchi when the lung tissue between these airways and chest wall is airless. The sound resembles that obtained by listening over the trachea. The expiratory sounds are generally more intense than inspiratory sounds and extend through greater part of the expiratory phase. Inspiratory sounds are moderately intense and do not extend throughout the inspiratory phase and there is a pause between the end of inspiration and start of expiration. The quality of sounds is hollow, harsh and high pitched.

Vocal resonance: It is the resonance of sounds in the chest made by the voice. Intensity and character of vocal resonance on each side of the chest over different areas of the lung is noted. The patient is asked to repeat the word one-one or ninety-nine while auscultation is being done.

Adventitious/added sounds: They can arise from either lung or pleura. Quality of the adventitious sounds can be dry or moist.

Lung Sounds

- *Dry sounds:* Known as rhonchi. They are continuous sounds produced by partial obstruction of respiratory passages. For example bronchitis, bronchial asthma or bronchospasm.
- *Moist sounds:* Known as rales (coarse crackles) or crepitations (fine crackles). They are discontinuous crackling sounds produced in the alveoli, bronchioles and bronchi. They indicate the presence of fluid secretion in the air sacs or tubes.

Pleural Sounds

The common adventitious sound arising in the pleural cavity is a friction sound or pleural rub characteristic of pleuritic pain (pleurisy) that becomes prominent during deep inspiration due to rubbing of inflamed surfaces of pleura against each other.

Questions

1. Enumerate the conditions in which:
   - Trachea deviates from the midline
   - Vocal resonance increases
   - Vocal resonance decreases
   - Rhonchi are heard
   - Crepitations are heard
   - Bronchial breathing is heard.
2. Differentiate between vocal resonance and vocal fremitus.
3. Define Cheyne-Stokes breathing. Name the physiological conditions resulting in Cheyne-Stokes breathing.

EXPERIMENT NO. 2

AIM: TO RECORD THE VITAL CAPACITY AND THE EFFECT OF POSTURE ON VITAL CAPACITY

Equipment Description

Simple Spirometer/Vitalograph

The simple spirometer/vitalograph consists of an outer container filled with water in which 6-litre capacity gas bell floats. The float is attached to a chain, which passes over a calibrated pulley bearing a spring-loaded indicator needle; the needle moves with the pulley. The gas bell is counterpoised and has very little inertia and friction. The inlet tube is corrugated rubber canvas bearing a mouthpiece and is attached to a pipe fitted at the bottom of the water container.

Procedure

- The subject is explained about the procedure.
- The gas bell is brought to the lowest position so that pointer needle indicates zero.
- The patient is asked to breathe normally for a few minutes.
- Then he is asked to inspire as deeply and fully as possible with nostrils closed (with his thumb and fingers or nose clip) and to expire with maximum effort into the mouthpiece held tightly between the lips.
- The gas bell moves up and the pointer on the pulley indicates the volume of expired air.
- This measures vital capacity, which should be noted in the sitting, standing and lying down position, in order to study the effect of posture.
- Three readings are noted at an interval of 5 minutes.
- Each of the volumes is noted and the reading for best effort is taken for interpretation.

Questions

1. Define vital capacity. Give normal values in males and females.
2. What are the physiological factors affecting vital capacity?

EXPERIMENT NO. 3

AIM: TO RECORD LUNG VOLUMES AND CAPACITIES USING CLOSED CIRCUIT SPIROMETRY WITH BENEDICT-ROTH APPARATUS

Equipment Description

Benedict-Roth Spirometer

It consists of a bell of 6-litre capacity, four speed recording unit, a kymograph, gearbox, and three stopcocks; one to serve as a water outlet and other two for oxygen and any other gas. The two-way stopcock is carried in an adjustable arm and fitted with mouthpiece via corrugated rubber tubing (Fig. 1, Plate 1)

Procedure

- The bell is filled with atmospheric air by lifting it and allowing the air to be drawn in. To ensure that the spirometer is leak-proof, the bell is slightly pressed while keeping the breathing tube closed.
- After cleaning the mouthpiece with antiseptic solution, it is placed in the mouth of the subject. Its edge plate is inserted between gums and teeth and the horizontal plates are clenched with teeth.
- The nostrils are closed with thumb and fingers and breathing is continued into atmosphere, till it becomes normal.
- After turning the valve of the mouthpiece and connecting to spirometer, the subject is asked to breathe normally for 30 seconds. The drum speed is kept at 20 revolutions per minute.
- The record for the tidal volume is obtained on the moving drum which shows inspiration as upward excursion and expiration as downward deflection.
- To record inspiratory reserve volume the subject is asked to breathe in maximally after a normal tidal inspiration, and is asked to exhale maximally after normal tidal expiration to note expiratory reserve volume.
- To record vital capacity, he is instructed to exhale maximally after maximal inspiration.
- To record FEV1, the subject exhales as forcefully and rapidly as possible after maximal inspiration, with the drum speed adjusted at a higher speed.
- To record maximum voluntary ventilation (MVV), a nose clip is attached to the patient, the mouthpiece is placed into the subjects' mouth and he is asked to breathe as rapidly and deeply as possible for 10 seconds.
- From the deflections recorded, the volume of air inhaled or exhaled in one minute is calculated.

Questions

1. Enumerate and define all lung volumes and capacities (static and dynamic) and give their normal values in adults in both sides.
2. From the sample record obtained calculate the following:
   i. Tidal volume
   ii. Inspiratory reserve volume
   iii. Expiratory reserve volume

   iv. Vital capacity
   v. Forced expiratory volume in one second (FEV1).
3. How do you differentiate between obstructive and restrictive lung disease? Give some examples of restrictive and obstructive diseases.
4. What is Maximum voluntary ventilation (MVV)?
5. Define Breathing reserve and Dyspnoea index.

EXPERIMENT NO. 4

AIM: TO RECORD RESPIRATORY MOVEMENTS BY STETHOGRAPHY

Equipment

Stethograph, Marey's tambour, Stopwatch, Kymograph and time marker or Physiograph.

Stethograph

It consists of corrugated rubber tubing, which has a side tube, and a chain attached. The side tube is connected to Marey's tambour, which has a lever with a pointer that records the movement. Whenever the corrugated rubber tube is stretched due to respiratory movements, there is an increase in the length of the tube and the mean radius remaining constant, an increase in volume of the air inside the tube is associated with a fall in pressure. This results in depression of the diaphragm of the Marey's tambour and its lever records a downstroke with each inspiration. The opposite occurs with expiratory phase.

Procedure

- The corrugated rubber tube is tied around the subject's chest, in the fourth intercostal space.
- The connecting pressure tube is joined to Marey's tambour, which is mounted alongwith time marker on the same stand and the two levers made to touch the kymograph drum in the same vertical line. Normal respiratory movements are recorded keeping the speed of the kymograph at 2.5 mm/sec.
- The normal tracing is first obtained for some duration of time. Then one of the variables as mentioned below is applied and its effect on respiratory movements is recorded by obtaining the tracing for some more duration of time.

The effect of following variables on respiratory movements is observed:

Cough

The subject is asked to cough voluntarily for one or two times and the effect is observed.

Speech

The subject is asked to speak out continuously for some duration and the effect is observed.

Deglutition

The subject is asked to swallow 2–3 sips of water while the respiratory movements are being recorded.

Hyperventilation

The subject is asked to breathe in and out as deeply and as fast as possible for 15–20 seconds and then let the breathing be spontaneous (without conscious effort) while the recording is going on continuously.

Breath Holding

The subject is asked to hold his breath during different phases of respiration while the normal recording is going on and breath holding time in each case is noted.

- After normal inspiration
- After normal expiration

- After deep inspiration
- After deep expiration.

Please note: A gap of 2–3 minutes should be given between each breath holding.

Exercise

- Few normal respiratory excursions are recorded.
- The drum is stopped and the stethograph is removed from its attachment to the Marey's tambor.
- The subject is asked to do exercise in the form of spot running while standing at the same place, for 2–3 minutes.
- The stethograph is quickly reconnected to Marey's tambour and the effect is recorded on the drum.

Precautions

1. Do not allow the subject to see the recordings during the experiment.
2. Subject should be allowed to hyperventilate for a short period only.

Questions

1. What is the principle of stethography?
2. Define breaking point. Enumerate the factors which delay the breaking point.
3. Comment upon your observations on respiratory movements following voluntary hyperventilation.

DEMONSTRATION NO. 1

AIM: TO RECORD PULMONARY FUNCTION TESTS WITH COMPUTERISED SPIROMETER

Equipment Description (Fig. 2, Plate 1)

Medspiror

Medspiror is a fibreglass cabinet, which houses the electronics, power supplies and operator controls. It is used with electromechanical pneumotach supplied with the instrument. The built in 40 column printer permits one or more printouts containing patient information, calculated, predicted and percentage predicted values of all the respiratory parameters, clinical interpretation of the results and two plots namely flow-volume curve and volume-time graph.

The Medspiror/Computerised Spirometer may be used to test the following parameters:

- FVC: Forced vital capacity
- FEV0.5: Forced expiratory volume in half second
- FEV1.0: Forced expiratory volume in first second
- FEV3.0: Forced expiratory volume in three seconds
- PEFR: Peak expiratory flow rate
- FEF25-75: Mean forced expiratory flow during the middle half of the FVC
- FEF2-12: Mean forced expiratory flow rate between 0.2–1.2 litres of volume change
- FEF 25%: Forced expiratory flow after 25% of the FVC has been expired
- FEF 50%: Forced expiratory flow after 50% of the FVC has been expired
- FEF 75%: Forced expiratory flow after 75% of the FVC has been expired
- FEV0.5 /FVC
- FEV1.0/FVC
- FEV3/FVC

  (FEV0.5/FVC, FEV1.0/FVC, FEV3/FVC:) Forced expiratory volume (timed) to forced vital capacity ratio expressed as percentage
- MVV: Maximal voluntary ventilation.

Procedure

To record the above parameters, Medspiror should be calibrated and the subject's data should be fed in.

To Record Forced Vital Capacity (FVC)

- A nose clip is attached to the patient and a clean mouthpiece is placed into the breathing tube.
- Maximum inspiration is performed.
- Mouthpiece is placed firmly into the mouth.
- Maximum expiration is performed.
- Mouthpiece is removed.
- Immediately before the patient begins the forced expiratory phase of the manoeuvre, the E key should be pressed.

To Record Maximal Voluntary Ventilation (MVV)

- Enter M to prepare for an MVV manoeuvre.
- Enter 2 digits to establish the number of seconds the MVV test is to be run (between 10–30 seconds). Generally it is performed for 10 seconds.
- A nose clip is attached to the patient, the mouthpiece is placed into the patient's mouth and the patient is instructed to breathe normally.
- With display reading 00 and the patient settled, he is asked to breathe as rapidly and deeply as possible.
- After the patient has begun the manoeuvre (one or two breaths), the E key is pushed, the display shows the number of seconds entered earlier.
- The display countsdown (in seconds) to 0 simultaneously as the patient performs the MVV test.

Computerised spirometers of different types can be used to measure different respiratory parameters using the same procedure as above with hardware/software settings in accordance with the type of instrument.

Questions

1. Name the conditions that affect the peak expiratory flow rate.
2. Explain maximal mid-expiratory flowrate (MMFR).
3. What is the clinical significance of timed vital capacity?

DEMONSTRATION NO. 2

AIM: TO DETERMINE BASAL METABOLIC RATE (BMR) IN A SUBJECT

Equipment

Benedict Roth apparatus and Oxygen cylinder.

Introduction

Basal metabolic rate refers to the minimum rate of energy expenditure under basal conditions that is compatible with life. It can be determined clinically by measuring the O_2 consumption of the subject in a resting state and is expressed as kcal/hour/m^2 body surface area (BSA).

Pre-requisites for Measuring Basal Metabolic Rate

- The subject should be kept fasting for 12–14 hours before the start of the test. This ensures that the subject is in post-absorptive state and the SDA of food does not affect BMR.
- He/she should be in a state of complete physical and mental rest at the time of the test. Physical rest is ensured by making the subject lie down on a comfortable couch and mental rest is ensured by providing him a relaxed, quiet atmosphere free from noise. Room temperature is adjusted in a comfortable range. The procedure is explained to the subject to clear any apprehensions regarding the experimental procedure.

Procedure

- The subject's age, sex, height and weight are noted.
- Barometric pressure and the temperature of the spirometer are measured.
- The subject is made to relax in the recumbent position for about half an hour before the commencement of the test.
- The calibrated spirometer chart is pasted on the drum of the spirometer and the inverted bell of the spirometer is filled with 100% O_2.
- The subject is asked to breathe in and out of the spirometer through the mouthpiece with nostrils clipped.
- The subject becomes familiarised with the breathing technique in few seconds after which the respiratory excursions are recorded on the moving drum of the Benedict-Roth apparatus for six minutes.
- As the O_2 in the bell gets consumed during respiration, the baseline of the respiratory tracing moves upwards
- The difference between the starting point and the end point of the baseline indicates the O_2 consumed during six minutes.
- The O_2 consumption in one hour is derived from this value.
- Caloric equivalents for 1 litre O_2 (kcal/h) are noted down after correction is done for temperature and barometric pressure from Mckesson chart.
- The body surface area (BSA) of the subject is calculated by using the Dubois body surface chart (printed on the back of BMR recording chart) or Dubois formula [BSA (m^2)= $W_{0.425} \times H_{0.725} \times 0.007184$].
- This gives O_2 consumption in Kcal/h/sq. m. body surface area, i.e. basal metabolic rate (BMR).
- Predicted BMR is obtained from the table of the Mckesson chart as per age and sex of the subject (also printed on the back of BMR recording chart).

- The percentage deviation of the obtained BMR from predicted BMR is calculated. A deviation of ±15% is considered to be within normal limits.

Normal Values of BMR in Adults

Males : 40 Kcal/h/m^2 body surface area.
Females : 37 Kcal/h/m^2 body surface area.

Question

1. Enumerate the factors that affect basal metabolic rate (BMR).

DEMONSTRATION NO. 3

AIM: TO DEMONSTRATE THE PROCEDURE OF CARDIOPULMONARY RESUSCITATION ON A SUBJECT

The cardiopulmonary resuscitation is an emergency life-saving procedure for a person presented with cardiorespiratory arrest.

Cardio-respiratory arrest is defined as the abrupt failure of the heart or respiration or both to maintain adequate cerebral blood flow.

It can be divided under two headings:
1. Artificial respiration
2. Cardiac massage.

Artificial Respiration

Mouth-to-Mouth Breathing

- The subject is positioned flat on the back and the neck is extended.
- The patency of his airways is checked and any obstructions if present are cleared.
- The nostrils are closed and his mouth is opened.
- A deep inspiration is taken by the examiner and the examiner's mouth is applied to the subject's mouth and forceful exhalation is done into the subject's mouth. The expansion of his chest is noted.
- A rate of 10–12 breaths per minute is maintained.

Cardiac Massage

- The heel of one hand is placed at the junction of upper 2/3rd and lower 1/3rd of the sternum and the heel of the other hand is kept over and parallel to the first.
- Keeping the elbows straight the pressure is exerted vertically downwards on to the sternum and the sternum is compressed by about 4–5 cm in each compression.
- Compressions should be maintained at a rate of 70–80 per minute.

If resuscitation is being done by one person only then a ratio of 15 compressions to two breaths should be maintained and if resuscitation is done by two persons then a ratio of 5 compressions to one breath should be maintained.

Other Methods of Artificial Respiration

Holger-Nielson Method

- Also called "*Back Pressure Arm Lift* "method.
- Subject is placed in prone position and his head is turned to one side.
- His arms are abducted at shoulders (in such a way that they lie at right angle to the trunk) and flexed at the elbow.
- The operator kneels down on one knee in front of the subjects' head with his other foot placed near the subjects' elbow.

- Now the subjects' arms are held just above the elbow, lifted and drawn upward in such a way that the chest gets expanded. This helps in inspiration.
- The arms of the subject are gently dropped.
- Hands of the operator are then placed on the back of the subject with fingers spread wide apart.
- The operator now sways forward, transmitting his weight on the back of the subject through his arms and hands. This promotes expiration.
- This cyclical procedure of arm lifting and then back pressure is performed at a rate of about twelve per minute.

Sylvester Method

- Also called "*Arm Lift Chest Pressure*" method.
- Steps are same as for Holger-Nielson method except that the subject is placed supine and pressure is applied on the chest wall to promote expiration instead of back pressure.
- This method has an advantage over Holger-Nielson method that cardiac massage can also be done.

Schafers Method

- The subject is placed in prone position and the pressure on the back is applied to aid in expiration, in the same manner as for the Holger-Nielson method.
- This method implies that the inspiration will follow the above manoeuvre due to elastic recoil of the chest wall.

Anaesthetic Machine

In patients of respiratory failure or those undergoing surgery under general anaesthesia, artificial respiration is given by anaesthetic machine through an endotracheal tube inserted into the trachea.

Tracheostomy

In patients not able to maintain their respiration due to obstruction in nasal and pharyngeal passages or those requiring surgeries of head and neck regions, an opening is created at the level of 3rd, 4th or 5th tracheal ring and trachea is intubated through this opening.

Questions

1. Mention the procedure for carrying out, cardiac and respiratory resuscitation simultaneously.
2. What is the method of cardiac massage in infants?
3. What is the use of defibrillator?
4. Name the different methods of artificial respiration.

Chapter 2

Cardiovascular System

EXPERIMENT NO. 1

AIM: TO EXAMINE THE CARDIOVASCULAR SYSTEM

Equipment

Stethoscope

Examination of cardiovascular system consists of:

- Examination of precordium
- Examination of arterial pulse
- Recording of blood pressure
- Examination of venous pulse.

General physical examination in relation to cardiovascular system should also be carried out before proceeding ahead, to look for important signs namely anaemia, cyanosis, clubbing, dyspnoea and oedema.

Examination of Precordium

It is done under four headings:

- Inspection
- Palpation
- Percussion
- Auscultation.

Inspection

Shape of the chest and precordium (area of chest wall overlying the heart) is inspected for symmetry, presence or absence of abnormal pulsations or engorged veins and apex beat. Position of apex beat is noted as a pulsation one centimeter internal to the mid-clavicular line in the fifth intercostal space.

Palpation

Apex beat: Palm of the hand is placed on the expected position of the apex beat and its precise location is noted using the finger.

Percussion

Percussion is done from the lungs towards the heart, to define the various borders of the heart. The pleximeter finger is kept parallel to the border defined. Detection of cardiac percussion boundary beyond the normal dullness indicates either enlargement of the heart or shift of the heart, due to disease.

Auscultation

Auscultation of the heart is done with the help of stethoscope, to hear the first and second heart sounds in various auscultatory areas. The third and fourth heart sounds are recorded with the help of phonocardiogram. Auscultation is done for abnormal heart sounds like murmurs, pericardial friction rub, etc.

- *Auscultatory areas of the heart*
  - *Mitral area:* Area overlying the apex beat. S_1 is heard better than S_2 and coincides with carotid pulse and apex beat.
  - *Tricuspid area:* This is the area just to the left and lower end of the sternum. S_1 and S_2 can be heard, S_1 better than S_2.
  - *Aortic area:* Area in the second intercostal space to the right of sternum. Both the S_1 and S_2 are heard but S_2 better than S_1.
  - *Pulmonary area:* It is the area in the second intercostal space to the left of the sternum. S_1 and S_2 are heard, S_2 is heard better than S_1 in some young individuals. The S_2 is split normally during inspiration.
- *Heart sounds*

  First heart sound (S_1):
  - Due to closure of A-V valves
  - Indicates start of ventricular systole
  - Sounds like "LUB"
  - Low pitch (25–45 Hz)
  - Longer duration (0.15 secs.).

  Second heart sound(S_2):
  - Due to closure of semilunar valves
  - Indicates onset of ventricular diastole
  - Sounds like "DUP"
  - High pitch (50Hz)
  - Shorter duration (0.12 secs.).

Examination of Arterial Pulse

(please also see page no. 51)

Arterial pulse can be examined in main peripheral arteries i.e. radial, brachial, femoral, popliteal and dorsalis pedis artery.

Radial artery is palpated more easily and hence preferred for the examination.

Arterial pulse can also be recorded with the help of a physiograph. After appropriate calibration, the transducer is tied around the pulp of the finger and pulse is recorded on running strip of paper.

Examination of the Jugular Venous Pulse

(please refer to page no. 37)

Recording of Blood Pressure

(please refer to page no. 41)

Questions

1. Name the conditions in which apex beat is shifted.
2. Name various cardiac areas and their significance.

EXPERIMENT NO. 2

AIM: TO EXAMINE THE JUGULAR VENOUS PRESSURE/JUGULAR VENOUS PULSE

The jugular venous pressure denotes mean pressure in internal jugular veins during cardiac cycle.

Procedure

- Clinically the jugular venous pressure is estimated by noting the upper limit of distension and pulsations of internal jugular veins with reference to the sternal angle. Examine the right internal jugular vein in good light with the subject reclining at an angle of 45 degrees. This angle is preferred as right atrium is assumed to be horizontal in this position. The neck is supported so that the neck muscles are relaxed.
- The jugular venous pulsations (2 or 3 per cardiac cycle) are visible at the right upper level of the blood column in the vein. The upper limit of normal jugular venous pressure is 2.5 cms above the sternal angle with the subject reclining at an angle of 45°. At this pressure, the jugular venous distension extends up to a point just below the clavicle and hence is not visible.
- The jugular venous pressure is given by the perpendicular height of the level of the venous pulsation above the sternal angle. Jugular venous pressure gives information about the mean right atrial pressure.
- The jugular venous pulse comprises of following 5 waves; 3 positive (ascents)—a, c, v wave and 2 negative (descents)—x, y
  - a wave—Due to atrial systole.
  - c wave—Due to bulging of tricuspid valve into right atrium during isovolumetric contraction phase.
  - v wave—Due to passive filling of atrium during ventricular systole against closed tricuspid valve.
  - x descent—Due to return of tricuspid valve ring back to original position when pulmonary valve opens.
  - y descent—Due to opening of tricuspid valve leading to ventricular filling.

Questions

1. Enumerate the conditions which lead to raised JVP.
2. How will you correlate different waves of JVP with those of ECG?

EXPERIMENT NO. 3

AIM: MEASUREMENT OF ARTERIAL BLOOD PRESSURE USING SPHYGMOMANOMETER

Definition

Blood pressure is defined as the force exerted by the moving column of blood against any unit area of vessel wall.

Blood pressure is almost always measured in mm of mercury, because the mercury manometer has been used as the standard reference for measuring blood pressure for many years. When we say that the pressure in a vessel is 60 mm of Hg, this means that the force exerted by the blood is sufficient to push a column of mercury up to a level of 60 mm.

Principle

It consists in balancing the air pressure against the pressure of blood in the brachial artery and then estimating the former by means of a mercury or aneroid manometer.

Methods of Measurement

Direct Method

Blood pressure can be measured directly by introducing a catheter into the artery. However, the procedure being invasive is not in common use.

Indirect Method

In 1896, Riva Rocci introduced a method for indirect measurement of blood pressure based on measuring the external pressure required to compress the brachial artery so that arterial pulsations could no longer be transmitted through the artery. The artery is occluded by wrapping an inflatable bladder which is encased in a non-distensible cuff, around the arm and inflating the bladder until the pressure in the cuff exceeds that in the artery. When the artery is occluded transmitted pulse waves can no longer be palpated or heard distal to the point of occlusion. As opening the valve on the inflation bulb reduces the pressure in the bladder, pulsatile blood flow reappears through the partially compressed artery, producing repetitive sounds generated by the pulsatile flow of blood.

Equipments

Sphygmomanometer or Aneroid Manometer, Stethoscope

Sphygmomanometer: It consists of a manometer with a calibrated scale for measuring pressure, an inflatable bladder in a cuff and an inflation-deflation device. Before any measurement is attempted the equipment must be checked to make sure that it is appropriate and in good order.

Manometer: The calibrated manometer reflects the pressure in the occluding cuff by the height of the column of mercury or by location of a rotating needle, on a dial scale. The mercury manometer is preferred and recommended over the aneroid manometer because it is more accurate, easier to maintain and less likely to get decalibrated.

Mercury column: The column of mercury in the top panel of the portable instrument has a height and a calibration scale from 0–300 mm of Hg, marked at intervals of 2 and 10 mm Hg. A steel reservoir containing mercury is attached to the calibrated mercury column made up of glass.

Inflation system: It consists of an inflatable bladder within a restrictive cloth sheath, an inflation bulb and connecting tubing. The cuff is applied by wrapping it completely around the limb so that non-inflatable portion overlaps that containing the bladder and is secured with a self-adhesive material such as velcro. Rubber tubing, which reflects the pressure inside the bladder, connects the bladder to the manometer. The bladder is also connected by a shorter tube to a rubber bulb with valve which is used to inflate and deflate the bladder at a rate controlled by the release valve.

Length and width of bladder: The length of bladder is one determinant of the area of pressure applied to the artery. If the bladder is too short, the blood pressure will be overestimated, since the pressure is not fully transmitted to the artery. The bladder should nearly or completely encircle the arm and the length should be at least 80% of the patient's upper arm length. The width of the bladder is 40% of the circumference of the upper arm at mid point. The width determines the length of the segment of artery to be occluded. British Hypertension Society has recommended the use of cuff with a dimension of 12.5 × 35 cms. Most of the commercial sphygmomanometers are provided with a cuff size of 12 × 22–26 cms.

Stethoscope

Laennec discovered stethoscope in 1819. It consists of a chest piece (diaphragm, bell), tubing and earpiece. It is placed over the occluded artery to amplify the sound.

Procedure

The purpose of the measurement should be explained to the subject in a reassuring manner and every effort made to put the subject at ease. The sequential steps for measuring the blood pressure in the upper extremity should include the following:

Palpatory Method

- The subject is seated in a quiet, calm environment with his or her bared arm resting on a standard table or other support so that the midpoint of the upper arm is at the level of the heart.
- The brachial artery is palpated and the cuff is placed in such a way that the midline of the bladder is over the arterial pulsation and then the cuff is wrapped snugly around the subject's bare upper arm. Avoid rolling up the sleeve in such a manner that it forms a tight tourniquet around the upper arm. Loose application of the cuff results in overestimation of the pressure. The lower edge of the cuff should be 2 cms above the antecubital fossa, where the diaphragm of the stethoscope is to be placed.
- The manometer is placed in such a way that the center of the mercury column or aneroid dial is at eye level and easily visible to the observer and the tubing from the cuff is unobstructed.
- The cuff is inflated rapidly to 70 mmHg and increased by 10 mmHg increments while palpating the radial pulse. The level of pressure at which the pulse disappears and subsequently reappears during deflation is noted. This procedure provides a necessary preliminary approximation of the systolic blood pressure to ensure an adequate level of inflation when the actual, auscultatory measurement is made. The palpatory method is particularly useful to avoid under-inflation of the cuff in patients with an auscultatory gap and over-inflation in those with very low blood pressure.

Auscultatory Method

- All the above steps are carried out before measuring the blood pressure by auscultatory method.
- The earpieces of the stethoscope are placed into the ear canals, angled forward to fit snugly.
- The diaphragm of the stethoscope is placed over the brachial artery pulsation, below the lower edge of the cuff, just medial to the insertion of biceps muscle. It is held firmly in place, making sure that the diaphragm makes contact with the skin around its entire circumference.
- The cuff is inflated rapidly and steadily to a pressure 20 to 30 mmHg above the level previously determined by palpation. The valve is partially unscrewed and the cuff is deflated slowly while listening for the appearance of the Korotkoff sounds.
- As the pressure in the cuff falls, the pressure level at the first appearance of clear, sharp and tapping sounds (phase I), at the abrupt muffling of these sounds (phase IV) and at the disappearance of sounds (phase V) is noted. The rate of deflation should be no more than 2 mm/pulse beat, during the period the Korotkoff sounds are audible, thereby compensating for both rapid and slow heart rates.
- After the Korotkoff sounds are no longer heard, the cuff is deflated slowly for at least another 10 mmHg to ensure that no further sounds are audible. The cuff is then deflated rapidly and completely and the subject is allowed to rest for at least 30 seconds.
- The systolic (phase I) and diastolic (phase V) pressures are immediately recorded and rounded off (upwards) to the nearest 2 mmHg. All values are recorded together with the name of the subject, the date and time of the measurement, the arm on which the measurement was made and the subject's position.
- The measurement should be repeated after at least 30 seconds and the two readings averaged.

Normal Average Values

Systolic: 100–140 mmHg
Diastolic: 60–90 mmHg.

Precautions

- Blood pressure should be recorded only after the person is relaxed and comfortable.
- In a nervous person first reading should be avoided as it is usually high and second reading is accurately representing the blood pressure.
- While tying the cuff, it should be kept in mind that cuff is not tied too tightly or too loose, because if the cuff is tied too tight it will give a lesser value as the artery is already compressed due to the tightness of the cuff. If it is tied too loose it will give a false high value.
- If successive readings have to be taken, the cuff pressure should never be kept high for longer period because it will cause reflex vasoconstriction in the peripheral vessel giving a false high reading.
- The arm should be horizontal and supported at the level of mid-sternum because dependency of the arm below the level of heart, leads to an overestimation of systolic and diastolic pressures of about 10 mmHg. Similarly, raising the arm above the level of the heart, leads to underestimation of these pressures.

Questions

1. Define systolic blood pressure, diastolic blood pressure, mean arterial pressure and pulse pressure.
2. What are Korotkoff's sounds and how they are produced?
3. What do you mean by auscultatory gap?

EXPERIMENT NO. 4

AIM: TO STUDY THE EFFECT OF POSTURE AND EXERCISE ON BLOOD PRESSURE

Equipments

Sphygmomanometer, Stethoscope

Effect of Posture

- The subject is allowed to lie comfortably on the couch in supine position for five minutes and the resting blood pressure is recorded by auscultatory method, with all precautions.
- The subject is then asked to stand and the blood pressure is recorded immediately after standing and 2 minutes after standing. This constitutes one set of recording.
- Three sets of such recordings are taken.

Inference

The experiment to find out the effect of change of posture on blood pressure indicates the integrity of cardiovascular reflex mechanisms. Sustained drop in systolic blood pressure by more than 20 mm Hg or diastolic blood pressure by more than 10 mm Hg after standing for at least 2 minutes indicates postural hypotension.

Effect of Isotonic Exercise

- The resting blood pressure is recorded in sitting/ lying down position.
- Keeping the cuff tied to the arm (disconnecting the mercury manometer) the subject is asked to perform any of the following exercises:
- To jog for 3–5 minutes on a jogger.
- To step up and down a Harvard step for 3–5 minutes.
- To hop on the floor lifting both feet together, 15–20 cm above the ground, for 3 min.
- The blood pressure is recorded immediately after exercise and then after every one minute till the resting values are achieved.
- The time taken for recovery is noted.

Effect of Isometric Exercise

This is done by handgrip test. Baseline blood pressure recordings (systolic as well as diastolic) are obtained. Using the handgrip dynamometer, the subject is asked to perform maximal voluntary contraction (MVC) and the maximum force exerted is noted down. After giving rest to the hand for a while, the subject is made to perform the same isometric exercise at 30% value of maximal force exerted for a maximum time up to 5 minutes or till such time that the subject is able to perform the exercise comfortably. Blood pressure is recorded every minute during the period of exercise. The response to the test is taken as the difference between the mean of 3 resting blood pressure recordings and the maximum reading of blood pressure during exercise (i.e. just before the release of handgrip).

Precautions

If at any stage, the subject feels discomfort in continuing the exercise, he should be asked to discontinue immediately.

Questions

1. What are the cardiovascular compensatory mechanisms to check the postural change in blood pressure?
2. What is orthostatic hypotension?
3. How isotonic and isometric exercises influence blood pressure?

EXPERIMENT NO. 5

AIM: CLINICAL EXAMINATION OF PULSE

Definition

Arterial pulse is defined as the rhythmic expansion of the arterial wall due to transmission of pressure waves along the walls of the arteries that are produced during each systole of the heart.

The pulse: The pulse wave has an upstroke and a downstroke. The percussion wave or tidal wave occurs due to ejection of blood from the ventricle during systole. The dicrotic wave occurs due to rebound of blood against the closed aortic valve during diastole. The dicrotic notch represents the closure of aortic valve. Sometimes, in the upstroke of the pulse wave, a small anacrotic wave is seen, which occurs due to change in the velocity of ejection of blood from the ventricle towards late systole.

Procedure

- Usually clinical examination of the pulse is done by palpating the radial artery.
- To feel the radial pulse easily, the forearm of the subject is semi pronated and the wrist is slightly flexed.
- The radial pulse is examined by compressing the radial artery against the head of the radius.
- Palpation is done by three fingers. The distal finger is used to apply pressure to prevent retrograde pulsation from the palmar arch, the proximal finger is used to vary the pressure to judge the force and tension of the pulse and the middle finger is used to feel the pulse wave.
- The following aspects of the pulse are studied:
  - i. Rate
  - ii. Rhythm
  - iii. Volume
  - iv. Character
  - v. Condition of the vessel wall
  - vi. Synchronicity
  - vii. Radiofemoral delay
  - viii. Pulse deficit
  - ix. Other peripheral pulses.

Rate: The three fingers are placed on the artery and the pulse is counted for one minute after the nervousness of the patient subsides, i.e. when the pulse resumes the normal rate. Normal rate varies from 60–90 beats per minute for an adult.

Rhythm: It is the spacing order at which successive pulse waves are felt. When spacing between all the waves is constant, the pulse is said to be regular. When the spacing is not constant the pulse is said to be irregular. The irregular pulse may have a fixed pattern of irregularity, i.e. regularly irregular or the irregularity may not have any pattern, i.e. irregularly irregular.

Volume: It is the degree of expansion of the arterial walls during each pulse wave. It is felt as an uplift given to the palpating fingers and compared bilaterally. Usually under physiological conditions, the volume is normal and equal on both sides.

Character: The character of a pulse is described as 'normal' when no abnormalities are detected in the rate, rhythm, volume and the waveform of the pulse. Under the heading character, rate of rise and fall of the pulse waveform is noted and it is better appreciated by recording the arterial pulse with a help of a transducer applied to the pulp of the finger. The transducer is connected to physiograph which records the arterial pulse on moving paper (Please *see* demonstration no. 1 for details).

Condition of the vessel wall: Place the three middle fingers on the artery to assess the condition of the arterial wall. Obliterate the flow of blood into the artery by pressing the index finger. Then palpate the artery with the middle finger. Roll the artery against the bone to assess the thickness of arterial wall. Normally the arterial wall is not palpable. But in old age it is well palpable.

Synchronicity: Compare all the features of the radial pulse on two sides by simultaneously palpating radial artery on both the sides. Under normal conditions all the features are same.

Radiofemoral delay: Compare the appearance of radial pulse with the appearance of the femoral pulse and note if any delay is present between the two. Normally there is no radiofemoral delay.

Pulse deficit: Heart rate is also simultaneously measured over the precordium by auscultation to detect any pulse deficit.

Other peripheral pulses: Palpate the temporal, carotid, brachial, femoral, popliteal, posterior tibial and dorsalis pedis arteries of both sides and see if the pulses are well felt and appear simultaneously on both sides.

Precautions

- The subject should rest and relax for a minimum of five minutes.
- The subject's arm should be semi-pronated and the wrist should be semi-flexed.
- Pulse rate should be calculated for a minimum of one minute.
- If the pulse rate is irregularly irregular, heartbeats must be auscultated simultaneously, to detect pulse deficit if present.
- Pulses of both the sides should be examined and compared.

Questions

1. Give reason for low pulse rate in athletes.
2. What do you understand by the following?
   a. Sinus arrhythmia
   b. Pulse deficit.
3. Enumerate the physiological and pathological causes of tachycardia.

EXPERIMENT NO. 6

AIM: TO PERFORM CARDIOVASCULAR ENDURANCE TESTS

Cardiovascular or aerobic fitness or cardiovascular endurance forms one of the most important components of physical fitness. It is an index to measure the amount of oxygen transported in the blood to the heart and pumped by the heart to the working muscles and the efficiency of the muscles to use oxygen. Increasing cardiovascular fitness means increasing the capability of the heart and the rest of the cardiovascular system in their important task, i.e. to supply oxygen and energy to our body.

Cardiovascular fitness is best improved by activities, which employ large muscle groups working dynamically. Such activities include walking, jogging, running, swimming, skating, cycling and stair climbing. All these activities promote isotonic muscular exercise.

Tests for Aerobic Fitness

There are numerous fitness tests for aerobic fitness ranging from sophisticated laboratory tests to simple field tests. They are all designed to quantitatively measure or predict maximal oxygen uptake (maximal aerobic power, VO_2max). Depending upon energy expended and oxygen utilisation during these tests, they can be divided into two categories: maximal tests and submaximal tests.

The most common maximal test procedures used for testing cardiovascular fitness are:

1. Maximal oxygen uptake tests (on a Treadmill or Bicycle ergometer)
2. Continuous run test for a fixed time or distance.

Stressing the body by exercising to exhaustion, as in the maximal tests, is not appropriate sometimes (especially in the elderly and those prone to coronary heart disease). Hence, the submaximal tests which impart less load on the cardiovascular system are recommended.

The most common submaximal test procedures used are:

- Step test (Harvard step test)
- Bicycle ergometer
- Walking test.

Harvard step test: The Harvard step test was developed by Harvard Fatigue laboratory and is conducted as follows:

- The subject steps up on to a standard gym bench (45 cm high) once every two seconds i.e. 30 steps/min for five minutes or until he can no longer maintain the rate of 30 steps/min for 15 sec. He is instructed to start with one foot (right or left) and use that same foot as the starting "step up" foot throughout the exercise.
- A metronome is used to maintain the stepping rate.
- The pulse is counted for 30 seconds, one minute after finishing the test—Pulse 1.
- Two minutes after finishing the test, the pulse is counted again for 30 seconds—Pulse 2.
- Three minutes after finishing the test, the pulse is counted for 30 seconds—Pulse 3.

Unnecessary movements and talking by the subject should be avoided when heart rates are being counted since any such activity can affect the heart rate and influence the results.

The change in heart rate at three different time intervals indicates the recovery time after exercise, i.e. how quickly the person's heart rate returns to baseline after exercise. The step test is based on the principle that a person with a higher fitness level will have a smaller increase in heart rate and faster recovery time.

Harvard Step Test Fitness Scoring

$$\frac{100 \times \text{test duration in seconds}}{2 \times \text{Total heart beat in the recovery period, i.e.}}$$

(Sum of pulse 1, pulse 2 and pulse 3)

The range of scores for the Harvard step test and the physical condition rating based on the score are as follows:

Step test score	Rating
>90	Excellent
80–89	Good
65–79	High average
55–64	Low average
<55	Poor

VO_2max Tests

VO_2max is the maximum amount of oxygen in ml, which can be consumed by a person in one minute/kg of body weight. A person with a higher VO_2max is considered to be fit and can exercise more intensely.

Factors Affecting VO_2max

a. Ability of muscular system to use oxygen in breaking down fuels.
b. Combined ability of cardiovascular and pulmonary systems to transport oxygen to the muscular system.

Maximum heart rate is the highest number of heart beats per minute when exercising maximally. It is calculated by using following formula (Bruce protocol).

$$\text{MHR} = 220 - \text{Age}$$

A person can increase his VO_2max by working out at an intensity that increases his heart rate between 65–85% of his maximum heart rate (MHR), for at least twenty minutes 3–5 times a week.

Procedure

Exercise is performed on an appropriate ergometer (treadmill, bicycle). The exercise workloads are selected to gradually progress in increments from moderate to maximal intensity. Oxygen uptake (VO_2max) is calculated from measures of oxygen or carbon dioxide in the expired air and minute ventilation and the maximal level is determined at or near test completion. The subject is considered to have reached his/her VO_2max if any of the following occur: (1) Volitional exhaustion, (2) A plateau or 'peaking over' in oxygen uptake, (3) Maximal heart rate is achieved.

Equipment

Oxygen and carbon dioxide analyzers, ergometer on which workload can be modified, stop watch. Expired air may be collected and volumes measured via Douglas bags or by pneumotach.

Bruce Treadmill Test[14]

To undertake this test we require:

- Treadmill where speed and grade of inclination can be adjusted
- Stop watch.

Procedure

The subject runs on a treadmill to exhaustion. At timed stages during the test the speed (km/hr) and grade of slope (%) of the treadmill are increased as detailed in the table below:

Stage	Time (min.)	Speed (km/hr)	Slope
1	0	2.74	10%
2	3	4.02	12%
3	6	5.47	14%
4	9	6.76	16%
5	12	8.05	18%
6	15	8.85	20%
7	18	9.65	22%
8	21	10.46	24%
9	24	11.26	26%
10	27	12.07	28%

The treadmill is set up with the stage 1 speed (2.74 km/hr) and grade of slope (10%) and the subject commences the test. At the appropriate times during the test the speed and slope of the treadmill are adjusted. After 3 minutes into the test the speed is adjusted to 4.02 km/hr and the slope to 12% and so on.

The stop watch is started at the start of the test and stopped when the subject is unable to continue and duration of the test is noted.

Analysis

From the total running time, VO_2max can be calculated as follows:

- VO_2max = (Time × 1.444) + 14.99

  'Time' is the total time of the test expressed in minutes and fractions of a minute.

  For example 13 minutes and 15 seconds means = 13.25 minutes. Hence VO_2max = (13.25 × 1.444) + 14.99 = 34.123 mL/kg/min.

  Interpretation of the VO_2max score can be done from the tables of VO_2max.

Questions

1. How do you derive target heart rate from Bruce protocol?
2. Define VO_2max. What is its significance?

DEMONSTRATION NO. 1

AIM: TO OBTAIN PULSE TRACING USING STUDENT'S PHYSIOGRAPH

Equipments

Student's Physiograph (Fig. 3, Plate 2), Pulse Transducer

Procedure

- The sensor is placed on the pulp of the finger
- The sensor is connected to the input of the coupler
- The speed of the physiograph is adjusted
- The position of the pen of the physiograph is also adjusted to get the recording at the centre of the paper
- 10–15 beats are recorded
- Recorded pulse wave has following components:
  P—*Percussion wave*: Due to rapid ejection phase of ventricular systole
  T—*Tidal wave*: Due to slow ejection phase of ventricular systole
  n—*Dicrotic notch*: Due to closure of aortic valves
  D—*Dicrotic wave*: Due to rebound of blood against closed aortic valve during diastole.

Questions

1. Define arterial pulse
2. Draw labelled diagrams of various abnormal pulse tracings.

DEMONSTRATION NO. 2

AIM: TO RECORD ELECTROCARDIOGRAM USING PORTABLE ECG MACHINE

Principle

It is the record of electrical activity generated by the heart with each heart beat, conducted through body fluids that act as volume conductors and picked up by surface electrodes placed at specific points.

For the bipolar recording the electrical potentials are recorded by two active electrodes, thus comparing the potential difference at two reference points at that particular instance.

For unipolar recording, the electrical potential is recorded between an active electrode (exploring) placed on the designated area of the body and other indifferent electrode (kept as zero potential) by connecting electrodes placed on right arm, left arm and left leg to a central terminal through 5000 ohms resistance.

Equipments

a. *Electrocardiograph:* It consists of a sensitive galvanometer with a stylus which gets heated up and inscribes on a thermosensitive graph paper (Fig. 4, Plate 2).
b. *Lead system (electrodes):* It consists of standard bipolar and unipolar limb leads and chest leads.
c. *Cardiac jelly:* It is used to reduce the skin resistance.

Placement of leads

1. *Bipolar limb leads:* These are placed in following Table.

Bipolar limb leads

Lead	Position	
	+ve	–ve
LI	Left arm	Right arm
LII	Left leg	Right arm
LIII	Left leg	Left arm

2. *Unipolar leads:* These are divided into limb leads and chest leads.
   i. *Augmented unipolar limb leads*: These are denoted by aVR, aVL and aVF and represent electrical activity of the cavity of ventricles, left upper side of heart and inferior surface of heart respectively.

Augmented unipolar limb leads

Lead	Position
aVR	Right arm
aVL	Left arm
aVF	Left foot

ii. *Unipolar chest leads*:

Unipolar chest leads

Lead	Position
V_1	4th intercostal space, right border of sternum
V_2	4th intercostal space, left border of sternum
V_3	Midway between V_2 and V_4
V_4	5th intercostal space in the midclavicular line
V_5	Anterior axillary line at the level of V_4
V_6	Midaxillary line at the level of V_4
V_7	Posterior axillary line at the level of V_4

- Another electrode is placed on right leg for grounding to minimize electrical interference.

Procedure

- The subject is made to lie down comfortably in supine position
- Jelly is applied at the points of contact of electrodes. Electrodes are connected
- The sensitivity is adjusted so that a vertical deflection of 10 mm is obtained by 1mv of potential generated
- Recording is done at a speed of 25 mm/sec.

Alternately, the ECG can also be recorded on a Physiograph.

Recording on Physiograph

Equipment Required

- Physiograph
- Limb leads
- Chest leads
- Biopotential coupler.

Procedure

- Coupler is plugged into the console with the console mains off.
- Physiograph is calibrated.
- Mode is set at ECG.
- 50Hz filter is put ON.
- Subject's skin is cleaned with spirit, gel is applied and electrodes are placed on the limbs and chest as per the conventional electrode placements.
- Electrodes for various leads are connected with 3 pin junction box and the junction box to the coupler.
- Paper is run using thumb screw.
- Records are taken for each lead.
- Record obtained is studied.

Question

1. Comment on the various wave forms and intervals of normal ECG.

DEMONSTRATION NO. 3

AIM: TO CALCULATE SYSTOLIC TIME INTERVALS (STI) FROM SIMULTANEOUSLY RECORDED TRACINGS OF ECG, CAROTID ARTERY PULSE AND HEART SOUNDS

Introduction

Determination of systolic time intervals is a non invasive technique and is done to assess the cardiac function, especially left ventricular performance. The determination of systolic time intervals includes left ventricular ejection time (LVET), pre-ejection period (PEP) and period of total electromechanical systole (QS2).

Equipments

Polyrite, ECG leads, phonotransducer, volume transducer with a pickup devices.

Procedure

- *For ECG recording:* Only single lead i.e. lead II (electrodes placed on right arm and left leg, left leg being positive) is used. This is connected to one channel of polyrite.
- *For carotid artery pulse recording:* Carotid artery is palpated in the neck at the medial border of sternocleidomastoid muscle, at the level of thyroid cartilage, with the help of thumb and a pick up device is placed over the site of maximum pulsation.
- This pick up device is connected to a volume transducer which in turn is connected to another channel of polyrite.
- *For recording heart sounds (phonocardiogram):* A phonotransducer is placed over the site of apex beat (one centimeter internal to the midclavicular line, in the fifth intercostal space, on left side).
- Subject is asked to lie down on a couch in supine position with body completely relaxed.
- Simultaneous recording of ECG, carotid pulse and heart sounds is done, taking care that the ink writing pens of all the channels are in line so that the tracings correlate with each other accurately.
- The tracings obtained are labelled.

Calculation of Systolic Time Intervals

- *Total electromechanical systole (QS2):* Period of total electromechanical systole (QS2) is calculated from the point at which a vertical line drawn from Q wave of ECG intersects the recording of first high frequency component of second heart sound (S2) on phonocardiogram. It includes electromechanical lag, isovolumic contraction time, pre-ejection period and left ventricular ejection time. Total electromechanical systole averages 546 milliseconds.
- *Left ventricular ejection time (LVET):* is calculated by marking the period between start of percussion wave (P wave) and the dicrotic notch in carotid pulse recording. It represents isotonic phase of left ventricular systole. It reflects the duration for which aortic valve remains open. It is directly related to stroke volume. Normal left ventricular ejection time averages 443 milliseconds.
- *Pre-ejection period (PEP):* A vertical line is drawn starting from Q wave of ECG. Pre-ejection period (PEP) is calculated from the point at which this line intersects the carotid pulse recording to the point

of start of percussion wave (P wave) in carotid pulse recording. It includes excitation-contraction coupling and isovolumetric contraction phase. PEP is obtained indirectly by subtracting LVET from QS2. Normal value of pre-ejection period averages 100 ± 13 milliseconds. A healthy ventricle has a short pre-ejection period and long ejection time. It is inversely related with stroke volume.

- *PEP/LVET ratio:* It is defined as ratio of pre-ejection period and left ventricular ejection time (PEP/LVET). It is the most reliable index of left ventricular systolic performance as it excludes other factors like age, sex, heart rate, stroke volume, etc. Normal value is 0.34 ± 0.04. The ratio depicts left ventricular ejection fraction. The ratio increases in heart failure, reduction in preload. Negative inotropic agents also increase this ratio.
- Systolic time intervals are affected by sympathetic activity and therefore should be corrected for heart rate by regression equation.

Question

1. Calculate different systolic time intervals from the graph obtained.

Chapter

3

Central Nervous System

EXPERIMENT NO. 1

AIM: TO PERFORM GENERAL NEUROLOGICAL EXAMINATION AND EXAMINATION OF HIGHER FUNCTIONS

Introduction

A routine examination of the whole nervous system is carried out in a sequential manner in order to exclude any major neurological disability. The nervous system examination is divided into following parts:

1. Examination of higher mental functions
2. Motor system examination
3. Sensory system examination
4. Examination of cranial nerves.

Brain is basically an input–output device. It receives its input via sensory system and produces action or output via motor system. These two systems are separately tested as defect in any modality can produce serious disease.

Examination of higher mental functions is performed to evaluate the intellect and cognition of the subject.

- In sensory system examination, we test for the sensation of touch, pressure, temperature, pain, stereognosis, vibration and proprioception.
- In motor system examination, the movement and strength, tone and bulk of muscles, reflexes, gait and involuntary movements of any group of muscles in the body are tested.
- In cranial nerve examination, 12 pairs of cranial nerves serving important sensory and motor functions essential for survival are tested bilaterally.

Examination of Higher Mental Functions

1. Consciousness
2. Orientation
3. General behaviour
4. Mood/affect

5. Delusion and hallucinations
6. Memory
7. Speech
8. General awareness and logical reasoning
9. Sleep and other normal daily functions.

Consciousness

Consciousness is a state of awareness of one's own self and one's environment. With altered states of consciousness ranging from stupor, semicoma and coma, the subject does not respond to various stimuli like visual, tactile, thermal and painful stimuli. Consciousness can be classified under various subheadings:

a. *Awake/alert:* Subject is conscious, active, awake and alert.
b. *Somnolence:* Subject can be awakened from his sleep by various stimuli and will make appropriate motor and verbal responses.
c. *Stupor:* Subject is aroused by painful and repeated stimuli and may respond to simple commands only for short periods. Restlessness and spontaneous movements might occur.
d. *Semi coma:* Painful stimuli cause withdrawal or other adaptive movements. Disorientation occurs.
e. *Coma:* Subject is deeply unconscious and does not respond to any kind of external stimulus or to inner need.

However, the Glasgow Coma Scale (GCS) is more specific in defining the altered states of consciousness (score of 3 represents worst and 15 represents the best score).

Orientation

Subject should be asked questions about time or day, date, month, year, the place where he is from, whom he is talking to and for how many days he has been in (if admitted). This elicits the orientation in time, person and place.

General Behaviour

The attire/dress of the subject, personal hygiene, the general attitude and cooperation with the examiner should be observed. It is noted whether he is evasive or hostile or shy or over frank. Note for any mannerisms or nervous behaviour.

Mood/Affect

The present mood of the subject is noted whether he is happy, euphoric, ecstatic, depressed, angry, having suicidal tendencies. Note whether the subject's mood is congruent with his speech and his general behaviour e.g. A subject describing the death of his mother in a euphoric mood suggests mental disease.

Delusions/Hallucinations

Delusions are false fixed beliefs, which cannot be changed despite evidence to the contrary. Hallucinations are false impressions from the organs of special senses (aural, visual and olfactory), for which no cause is found. The subject is asked whether he is having any hallucination and judge whether he is having any delusions.

Memory

Memory is defined as the retention and storage of acquired information in various areas of brain. The ability of the subject to recall various events is tested for the following three types of memory :

- Immediate
- Recent or short term memory
- Remote or long term memory.

The subject is asked to repeat a 7-digit number to test his immediate memory. For recent memory, the subject is asked to enumerate the contents of his breakfast or the news he has read in the morning.
To test for remote memory, the subject is asked about the date of his marriage or some significant life event in the past.

Speech

Speech abnormalities can be of two types:
a. Difficulty in articulation i.e. *dysarthria*
b. Disability in production of speech i.e. *aphasia*
In dysarthria, the speech can be *stammering/lalling* speech
In aphasia, there is disturbance of the ability to use language in speaking, writing or comprehending. It is further of three types:
a. *Fluent aphasia*
b. *Anomic aphasia*
c. *Non-fluent aphasia*
The classification of aphasias given above is based upon the site of lesion i.e.

- Wernicke's area or in arcuate fasciculus or in area 40, 41, 42 of auditory cortex (fluent aphasia)
- Broca's area (non-fluent aphasia)
- Angular gyrus (anomic aphasia).

Tests of Aphasia

Fluent Aphasia

- Lesion in Wernicke's area: The subject is asked or is presented with written words. He is unable to comprehend the meaning of spoken or written words. His speech is fluent but full of jargon or neologisms.
- Lesion in arcuate fasciculus: Also known as "*conduction aphasia*". The subject is asked about his name. He hears and understands and has good auditory comprehension but cannot put parts of the words together and thus cannot reply.

Anomic Aphasia

- Lesion in angular gyrus: Lesion in the angular gyrus in the categorical hemisphere leads to "*anomic aphasia*". The subject cannot understand written language or pictures as the visual information is not processed and transmitted to Wernicke's area.

Non-fluent Aphasia

- Lesion in Broca's area: The speech of the subject is slow and words are hard to come by. His speech is limited only to two or three words to express the whole range of meaning and emotion.
  1. *Spoken*: Patients is asked about his name. He hears and understands and knows what to reply but is unable to plan the precise order in which muscles have to be employed and thus cannot reply though he can give affirmation by nodding.
  2. *Written*: In a similar way, when a question is written, the subject can see and interpret it but fails to write a reply. But if a leading question is put, he can write yes or no correctly.

     In *motor aphasia*, the subject can comprehend the speech but cannot speak because of defect in productive mechanism i.e. Broca's area.

General Awareness and Logical Reasoning

The subject is asked some important questions about general awareness like who is the Prime Minister of our country. The subject is asked to repetitively subtract 5 from 100 to note his logical reasoning.

Sleep

The subject is asked about his sleep hours, any waking up during night, any desire to sleep in daytime or other problems. Sleep is disturbed in states of anxiety and some sleep disorders.

Questions

1. Define different types of memory.
2. What are the various altered states of consciousness?

EXPERIMENT NO. 2

AIM: EXAMINATION OF CRANIAL NERVES I-VI

Ist (Olfactory) Nerve

It is a pure sensory nerve concerned with olfaction. The subject is asked to find out by smelling only (keeping the eyes closed), familiar substances like clove oil, oil of peppermint, asafoetida or common bed side substances like soap, fruit, etc. put in small test tubes. Substances like ammonia should be avoided, as it irritates Vth cranial nerve also. The testing should be done in both nostrils separately (when testing through right nostril the subject is asked to block the left nostril and vice versa).

The complaints of any cough, cold or nasal blockage should be ruled out.

Observation

The subject should be able to identify the normal smell.

Anosmia (complete absence of smell), *parosmia* (alteration in the character of smell) or *hyposmia* (reduction in the sense of smell) should be looked for.

IInd (Optic) Nerve

It is a pure sensory nerve, subserving vision in all its faculties like light, form and colour sense. Each eye is separately tested for the following:

1. Visual acuity (Experiment no. 8)
2. Colour vision (Experiment no. 9)
3. Field of vision (Experiment no. 10).

IIIrd (Oculomotor) Nerve

It supplies

i. Ciliary muscle (helps in accommodation)
ii. Sphincter pupillae (helps in papillary constriction)
iii. Levator palpebrae superioris (elevation of upper eyelid)
iv. Extraocular muscles except superior oblique and lateral rectus.

IVth (Trochlear) Nerve

It supplies superior oblique muscle.

VIth (Abducens) Nerve

It supplies lateral rectus muscle.

Cranial nerves III, IV and VI are mixed nerves and are tested together as they innervate the extra ocular muscles which are responsible for the movements of the eyeball.

Examination of III, IV and VI Nerves:

1. The subject is made to sit comfortably. The eyes are observed for the following :
   a. Presence of ptosis—Drooping of upper eyelid.
   b. Lid lag in either eye—When patient is asked to look downward; the upper eyelid lags behind the eyeball.

   c. Presence of any squint or strabismus—An abnormality of ocular movements in which the visual axes do not meet at the point of fixation leading to *diplopia* or *double vision*.
   d. Presence of nystagmus—The involuntary rhythmic oscillations of eyeballs, when gaze is fixed in one direction.
2. *Examination of the eye movements in all directions:* Eye movements are tested by asking the subject to follow the movements of examiner's finger in upward, downward, medial, lateral and oblique directions. Following movements are looked for:
   a. Abduction—A function of lateral rectus.
   b. Adduction—A function of medial rectus.
   c. Elevation in full abduction—A function of superior rectus.
   d. Elevation in full adduction—A function of inferior oblique (rotates the eyeball outwards and pulls it upwards.
   e. Depression in full abduction—A function of inferior rectus.
   f. Depression in full adduction—A function of superior oblique (rotates the eyeball inwards and pulls it downwards).
3. *Examination of pupil*
   a. Size of pupil: Size of both the pupils is compared
   b. Shape of pupil: The shape of the pupil is noted, whether circular in outline (normal) or irregular
   c. Pupillary reflexes:
      i. *Light reflex*
         - *Direct light reflex*: Each eye is separately examined with the subject seated in shade or indirectly illuminated place with the other eye covered. He is asked to look at a distant object so that the accommodation is relaxed. A bright light is brought from the side and is shone into the eye to be tested.
           Observations: Immediate constriction of the pupil in the same eye.
         - *Indirect/consensual light reflex*: A hand is placed between the two eyes and light is thrown into one eye while the effect is observed on the other eye.
           Observations: Pupillary constriction in the unstimulated eye.
      ii. *Accommodation reflex*:
         The examiner's index finger is kept close to the subject's nose while the subject is asked to look at a distant object. Then the subject is asked to look at examiner's index finger quickly.

   The accommodation reflex comprises of three events:
   a. Constriction of pupil
   b. Convergence of the eyes
   c. Increase in the convexity (anterior curvature) of the lens.

Vth (Trigeminal) Nerve

It is a mixed nerve with sensory and motor functions. It is formed by three divisions:
1. Ophthalmic
2. Maxillary
3. Mandibular.

Testing of Motor Functions

a. The subject is asked to clench the teeth tightly and the hardness of *masseter* and *temporalis muscle* is tested on either side.
   Observations: The muscle on affected side fails to become prominent.
b. The subject is asked to open the mouth and jaw symmetry is noted.
   Observations: Any deviation of jaw indicates weakness of that part.

Testing of Sensory Functions

a. Touch, pressure, pain and temperature sensations are tested over the skin and mucous membrane of the face supplied by the three branches of trigeminal nerve.
b. Corneal reflex is tested by touching the lateral edge of cornea at its conjunctival margin with a wisp of cotton wool and reflex blinking of the eye is noted.

Questions

1. Comment briefly upon the following:
   a. Accommodation reflex
   b. Light reflex
   c. Argyll-Robertson pupil.

EXPERIMENT NO. 3

AIM: EXAMINATION OF CRANIAL NERVES VII – XII

VIIth (Facial) Nerve

It is a mixed nerve and consists of motor and sensory fibres.

Testing of Facial Nerve

1. The subject is seated comfortably and the face is observed for the following features:
   a. Expression of the face
   b. Depth of nasolabial folds
   c. Furrows on forehead
   d. Width of palpebral fissure
   e. Symmetry of angles of mouth.
2. *Testing of upper face:*
   i. The subject is asked to frown or look upwards and normal symmetrical wrinkling of the forehead is noted.
   ii. The subject is asked to shut his eyes as tightly as he can and normal descent of upper lids and rolling in of eye lashes is looked for.
   iii. The subject is asked to shut his eyes tightly and examiner tries to open them. Normally eyes cannot be opened while resistance is being applied by the subject.

   Bells's phenomenon: Rolling of eyeballs upwards during attempted forced eye closure. It is a normal phenomenon but is more obvious when eye closure is not possible in facial nerve palsy.
3. *Testing of lower face*:
   i. The subject is asked to whistle which is not possible in facial nerve palsy.
   ii. The subject is asked to show his teeth and the position of angle of mouth is noted. The mouth is deviated to a healthy side in facial nerve palsy because of unopposed action of muscle on healthy side.
   iii. The subject is asked to inflate his mouth with air and blow out his cheeks. Now, either side of cheek is gently tapped with a finger. The air leaks out from the affected side in facial nerve palsy.
   iv. The taste sensation from anterior two-third of the tongue is tested for sweet, salt and sour preparation.

   Facial nerve palsy can be divided into supranuclear and infranuclear palsy.

Supranuclear palsy: Lesion is above the facial nerve nucleus. Lower part of the face is mainly affected because the parts of the facial nuclei innervating the upper face are bilaterally innervated and therefore only partial paralysis of upper part of the face occurs. Taste sensation is spared.

Infranuclear palsy: Lesion is at the level or below the level of facial nerve nucleus. Both the upper and lower part of the face is affected because of damage to final common path i.e. facial nerve. There is loss of taste sensation from anterior 2/3rd of the tongue and *"hyperacusis"* (sounds on the side of the facial nerve palsy may seem unusually loud) because of the paralysis of stapedius muscle on the affected side.

VIIIth (Vestibulocochlear) Nerve

It is a pure sensory nerve and has two sets of fibres performing auditory and vestibular functions

1. Auditory Functions

a. Hearing tests or tuning fork tests (Experiment no. 11)
b. Audiometry.

2. Vestibular functions:

a. The subject is asked about any complaints of giddiness/dizziness and vertigo (external objects seem to move around the subject).
b. The subject is enquired for any history of *nystagmus* (involuntary rhythmic jerky movements of the eyeball).
c. *Romberg's sign*—This is a test for loss of position sense (sensory ataxia). The subject is asked to stand with his feet close together and is then asked to close his eyes. Romberg's sign is positive if he sways about or falls to either side on closing his eyes.

IXth (Glossopharyngeal) Nerve

It is a mixed nerve consisting of motor and sensory fibres.

1. *Taste sensation:* Sensation of taste on posterior one-third of tongue is tested
2. *Palatal reflex:* The back of pharynx is tickled with a cotton wick and reflex contraction of pharynx is noted.

Xth (Vagus) Nerve

1. Tests for the palate

a. The subject is asked about any history of *regurgitation* of fluids through the nose during swallowing
b. Any nasal twang is noted
c. Palatal reflex is tested
d. The subject is asked to say 'Ah' and movement of both sides of palatal arch is observed.

2. Tests for the Larynx

Laryngoscopy i.e. direct visualization of vocal cords is done .

XIth (Accessory) Nerve

The size, shape and strength of trapezius and sternocleidomastoid muscles are evaluated.

Testing of trapezius muscle: The subject is asked to shrug his shoulders while the examiner presses them downwards.

Testing of sternocleidomastoid muscle: The subject is asked to rotate his head to one side, against the resistance applied by the examiner from contralateral side.

XIIth (Hypoglossal) Nerve

The tongue of the subject is inspected while at rest and while protruding from the mouth

1. Fasciculation/tremor is observed in relaxed tongue.
2. The subject is asked to protrude his tongue as far as possible and any deviation from midline is looked for.

3. To test the strength of muscles of the tongue of the subject is asked to push the tongue against the cheek as the resistance is applied with an index finger by the examiner.

Questions

1. Differentiate between Supranuclear and Infranuclear lesions of facial nerve.
2. What is the sensory innervation of the tongue?
3. What are the different modalities of taste and how do you test them? Which are the different areas of the tongue representing different modalities of taste?

EXPERIMENT NO. 4

AIM: TO ELICIT SUPERFICIAL REFLEXES

Definition

Superficial reflexes are the reflex contractions of the underlying muscles when superficial structures of body like skin and mucous membrane are stimulated. These are the polysynaptic reflexes.

Following superficial reflexes can be elicited

1. Plantar reflex
2. Abdominal reflex
3. Cremasteric reflex
4. Corneal reflex
5. Conjunctival reflex
6. Scapular reflex.

Plantar Reflex (L_5, S_1)

The outer edge of the sole of the foot is stimulated with a key or a stick by gentle scratching starting from the heel and moving towards the little toe along the lateral border of heel and then medially towards the great toe.

Normal response: Plantar flexion of toes.

Babinski's response/sign: Dorsiflexion of great toe and fanning of other toes.

Cause/reason: Occurs in upper motor neuron lesions.

Babinski's response occurs normally also in infants and in deep sleep.

Abdominal Reflex (T_7–T_{12})

The abdominal wall is stimulated with the help of a key or a wooden stick which is passed across the abdominal skin from the outer aspect towards midline in the plane of the dermatome.

Normal response: Contraction of underlying abdominal musculature.

This reflex is difficult to observe in obese/anxious persons.

Cremasteric Reflex (L_1, L_2)

The upper and inner aspect of thigh is gently stroked from above downwards with a blunt object.

Normal response: Elevation of testicles on the side of stimulation due to contraction of cremasteric muscle.

Corneal Reflex (Cranial Nerve V and VII)

The lateral edge of cornea is touched at its conjunctival margin with the wisp of cotton wool from the lateral side of the eye (outer canthus) while the subject is asked to look directly in front.

Normal response: Blinking (Bilateral).

Conjunctival Reflex (Cranial Nerve V and VII)

The bulbar conjunctiva is touched with the wisp of cotton wool.

Normal response: Blinking (Bilateral).

Scapular Reflex (C_5–T_1)

The inter scapular region is stimulated with a blunt object.

Normal response: Contraction of scapular muscles.

Question

1. What do you understand by Babinski's response?

EXPERIMENT NO. 5

AIM: TO ELICIT DEEP REFLEXES

Definition

Reflex is an involuntary response to adequate sensory stimulus and depends upon the integrity of reflex arc.

Deep reflexes can be elicited by providing a stimulus, which is, sudden stretching due to single sharp tap on the tendon of a lightly stretched muscle. The reflex is integrated at the spinal cord level but is modified by the activity of the higher centres through descending pathways.

The following deep reflexes are elicited:

1. Knee jerk
2. Ankle jerk
3. Biceps jerk
4. Triceps jerk
5. Supinator jerk
6. Jaw jerk.

Gradation of response: The muscle contraction or movement of the joint is noted and the response is graded as follows:

0. Absent
1. Present
2. Brisk
3. Very brisk
4. Clonus.

Jendrassik's Manoeuvre

When reflexes are feeble reinforcement can be done by asking the subject to make a strong voluntary effort by hooking the fingers of two hands together and then pulling them apart as hard as possible or to make a fist with the ipsilateral hand. The reinforcement helps by increasing the γ-discharge thereby increasing the sensitivity of muscle spindle to stretch.

Knee Jerk (L_2–L_4)

This can be elicited in two positions

- Sitting.
- Supine.
- *Knee jerk in sitting position:* When the subject is sitting at the edge of the bed or chair with legs hanging freely over the edge, he is asked to cross one leg over other. Then a sharp tap is given on the patellar tendon after palpating it.
- *Knee jerk in supine position:* The patient's legs are kept in semiflexed position and the hand is placed underneath the knee to be tested so as to raise it off the bed and let it completely rest on the examiner's arm. The patellar tendon is struck with the hammer.

Observation

Extension of the knee due to contraction of the quadriceps femoris muscle.

Ankle Jerk (S_1, S_2)

The lower limb is placed on the bed, everted and slightly flexed. The foot is slightly dorsiflexed with one hand so as to stretch the Achilles tendon and with the other hand, the tendon is struck on its posterior aspect.

Observation: Plantar flexion of foot due to contraction of the calf muscle.

Clonus: It is the exaggerated response of the muscle to sustained stretch, manifested through alternate contraction and relaxation of the muscle.

Physiological basis of clonus: Activation of stretch—Inverse stretch reflex.

Ankle clonus: The subject is made to lie down. The knee is bent slightly while supporting with one hand. The foot is grasped with the other hand and briskly dorsiflexed and sustained.

Observation: Repeated alternate flexion and extension of foot called clonus is observed.

Biceps Jerk (C_5, C_6)

The elbow is flexed at right angle and the forearm is placed in semipronated position. The biceps tendon is struck by placing the thumb or index finger on it.

Observation: Contraction of the biceps muscle leading to flexion and slight pronation of forearm.

Triceps Jerk (C_6, C_7)

The elbow is flexed and the forearm is allowed to rest across the subject's chest. The triceps tendon is palpated and struck just above the olecranon process.

Observation: Extension of the forearm with contraction of triceps muscle.

Supinator Jerk (C_5, C_6)

The elbow is placed slightly flexed and slightly pronated. Then a sharp tap is given on the supinator tendon over the styloid process of radius.

Observation: Supination of the elbow.

Jaw Jerk (Trigeminal Nerve Nuclei)

The subject is asked to keep the mouth slightly open. The finger is kept over the chin and is tapped suddenly with the finger of other hand.

Observation: Closure of jaw.

Precautions

- The subject is asked to be completely relaxed
- Adequate tension in the muscle is obtained by passively stretching and supporting the limb
- The portion of limb where the contraction of the muscle is to be elicited is exposed
- A soft rubber percussion hammer is used to give sharp blow on the tendon.

Questions

1. Define clonus.
2. Explain the physiological basis of Jendrassik's manoeuvre.

EXPERIMENT NO. 6

AIM: TO PERFORM EXAMINATION OF THE MOTOR SYSTEM

Introduction

The impulses from the motor precentral gyrus and other regulatory areas of the cerebral cortex travel via the

1. Upper motor neurons
2. Lower motor neurons.

Upper Motor Neuron (UMN)

Corona radiata emanates from the precentral gyrus and converges onto the internal capsule and passes through cerebral peduncle of the mid brain. Further it gets dispersed in the pons and reunites to form the pyramid at upper end of the medulla. Crossing over of the fibres occurs here to opposite side of lower medulla after which the fibres descend in the respective lateral columns of the spinal cord. The fibres end in the anterior horn cells located in the grey matter of spinal cord.

The neurons travelling from precentral gyrus to the anterior horn cell are known as upper motor neurons.

Lower Motor Neuron (LMN)

It carries the information supplied by the upper motor neuron to the motor end plate. The motor fibres arise from the anterior horn cells of spinal cord or from the cranial nerve nuclei in the brainstem. The motor fibres emerge through anterior nerve root to end on the motor end plate through the peripheral nerve. Muscular movements depend upon the integrity of lower motor neuron. If the final pathway is interrupted, weakness, *fasciculations*, muscle wasting, loss of tendon reflexes and hypotonia develop.

Postural movements and muscle tone depends on the neural activity in higher centres especially in corticospinal tract, extrapyramidal system and cerebellum. These activities can only reach muscle if the final pathway is intact.

In motor system examination, the following aspects of motor functions are tested:

1. Movement and strength or power of the muscles
2. Bulk of muscles
3. Tone of muscles
4. Reflexes
5. Gait
6. Involuntary movements.

Movement and Strength of Muscle

Muscle strength can be tested by two methods:

1. *Active method:* Subject moves the limb to be tested actively, while the examiner offers resistance against the movement.
2. *Passive method:* Muscle to be tested is put in a particular position and the subject is asked to hold the muscle in that position while an effort is made by the examiner to move it.

Following group of muscles are tested:

Main Flexors and Extensors

1. Shoulder girdle (flexion, extension, adduction, abduction and circumduction)

2. Upper arm muscles (flexion and extension of elbow mainly)
3. Forearm muscles (flexion, extension of wrist, pronation and supination of forearm)
4. Finger movements (flexion, extension, abduction and adduction)
5. Abdominal muscles—Tested by head raising and leg raising in supine position
6. Hip girdle (flexion, extension, abduction, adduction, medial and lateral rotation)
7. Thigh muscles (extension and flexion of the knee)
8. Leg muscles (dorsiflexion, plantar flexion, eversion and inversion of foot)
9. Muscles of the foot (dorsiflexion and plantar flexion, adduction and abduction of toes).

   *Grading of muscle power is done as follows:

   Grade 0: Complete paralysis

   Grade 1: A flicker of contraction only

   Grade 2: Power detectable only when gravity is excluded by appropriate postural adjustment

   Grade 3: The limb can be held against the force of gravity but not against the examiner's resistance

   Grade 4: There is some degree of weakness, usually described as poor, fair or moderate strength

   Grade 5: Normal power is present.

Nutrition/Bulk of Muscle

Procedure

Bulk of muscle varies with age, sex, body build and physical training. It is judged by inspection, palpation and by measuring circumference of the limbs with a measuring tape.

Muscle bulk is estimated in all the four limbs and also compared on corresponding sides. Muscle bulk can be:

- Normal
- Atrophied
- Hypertrophied

Flabby muscles indicate atrophy and hard muscles of abnormal shape indicate hypertrophy.

1. Measurement of muscle bulk in upper limb is done by measuring circumference 5 inches above the elbow joint and 4 inches below the elbow joint.
2. In lower extremity, the circumference 9 inches above the knee joint and 6 inches below the knee joint is noted.

Tone of Muscles

Tone of muscle is defined as a maintained partial state of contraction/tension in a healthy muscle at rest.

Hypertonia: Increase in the tone of the muscle

Hypotonia: Decrease in the tone of the muscle.

Procedure

- The subject is asked to completely relax his body while lying supine/sitting.
- Tone is tested by making passive movements at various joints (in upper limb : wrist, elbow and shoulder joint, and in lower limb : ankle, knee and hip joint) and resistance offered to the passive movements is noted.

**Source*: Medical Research Council Scale, Hutchison's Clinical Methods, Ref. No. 11

Reflexes

Please refer to experiment no. 4 and 5.

Coordination of Movements

It is the coordinated contraction and relaxation of different group of muscles in order to perform a purposeful motor task.

Coordination depends upon

1. Afferents—From muscle and joint receptors
2. Integrity of dorsal column
3. Vestibular system—Orientation of the body in space
4. Cerebellar system—Maintains smooth and balanced flow of impulses to muscles
5. Corticospinal tract function
6. Integrity of the other extrapyramidal areas of the cerebral cortex.

Coordination should be Tested in both Upper and Lower Limbs

1. *Upper limb:*
   i. The subject is asked to touch the tip of the nose with the tip of the right and left index fingers alternately first with eyes open and then with closed eyes (finger-nose test).
   ii. The subject is asked to touch the tip of one index finger to that of the examiner.
   iii. The subject is asked to rapidly supinate and pronate the forearm after flexing the elbow.
2. *Lower limb:*
   i. The subject is asked to walk along a straight line.
   ii. *Heel Knee test*: The subject is asked to place the heel of one foot on the opposite knee and then move it along the shin, first with his eyes open and then with eyes closed.
   iii. *Romberg's test*: The patient is asked to stand with his feet close together and his eyes open and then asked to close eyes . If the patient sways or falls with closed eyes, *Romberg's test* is positive and coordination is absent (*sensory ataxia*) [*in cerebellar ataxia a person sways with both open and closed eyes*].

Gait

Gait is observed by asking the subject to move freely in the room, to walk along a straight line, bare feet and to turn through 180 degrees quickly without losing balance. While looking for the cause of abnormal gait, local causes like osteoarthritis of the hip joint or any type of injury of the lower limb should be excluded. Following types of abnormal gait can be observed

- *Spastic gait*—Occurs in spinal cord diseases affecting corticospinal tracts
- *Drunken gait*—Occurs in cerebellar ataxia
- *Festinant gait*—Occurs in Parkinson's disease
- *Stamping gait*—Occurs in sensory ataxia
- *Waddling gait*—Occurs in myopathies and muscular dystrophies affecting proximal pelvic girdle muscles.

Involuntary Movements

Involuntary, unintended movements occur in different diseases of the nervous system and can occur at rest or superimposed on voluntary movements. Few clinically important involuntary movements are:

1. *Tremors:* These are the regular or irregular distal movements having an oscillatory character. They are classified as:
   - Fine, rapid tremors—Occur in anxiety, thyrotoxicosis
   - Resting tremors—Occur in Parkinson's disease
   - Intentional tremors—Occur in cerebellar disease
   - Coarse and irregular tremors—Also known as essential tremors—Senile tremors
   - Hysterical tremors—Characteristically worsened by examiners attempt to control them.
2. *Athetosis:* These are complex involuntary, writhing movements, usually more pronounced in distal muscles and are most commonly due to lesions of basal ganglia.
3. *Chorea:* These are rapid, irregular, involuntary dancing movements most commonly due to lesions of basal ganglia.
4. *Ballism:* These are involuntary movements that are flailing, intense and violent most commonly due to lesions of basal ganglia.
5. *Tics:* These are simple normal movements which become repeated unnecessarily to a point that they become an embarrassment. Common example is head nodding.
6. *Myoclonus:* These are rapid usually irregular, jerky movements of a group of muscles in a limb or even of the whole body often occurring due to an extraneous stimulus such as a sudden loud noise.

Questions

1. Differentiate between upper motor neuron and lower motor neuron lesions.
2. Enumerate the tests for cerebellar functions.
3. Define tremors and give etiological factors causing tremors.

EXPERIMENT NO. 7

AIM: TO EXAMINE THE SENSORY SYSTEM OF A SUBJECT

Introduction

Sensations can be divided into superficial (arising from the skin) and deep sensations (arising from somatic structures below the skin).

Before starting any procedure the nature of the test to be performed should be explained to the subject so as to get his full cooperation. The eyes should be closed for the different types of sensations tested. Corresponding points on both sides of the body should always be compared.

There are six main sensory modalities which can be tested:

1. Tactile sensibility (includes light touch, pressure, tactile localization and tactile discrimination)
2. Position sense
3. Stereognosis
4. Vibration sense
5. Pain
6. Temperature.

Tactile Sensibility

a. *Light touch:* A wisp of cotton wool is gently touched on different parts of the body and the subject is asked to say 'yes' every time he feels the touch.
b. *Pressure:* Pressure is defined as sustained touch. It is tested by applying pressure over the skin with a fingertip or the blunt end of a pencil.
c. *Tactile localisation:* It is the ability to tell precisely, the portion of the body part that is touched. The wisp of the cotton wool is touched on different parts of the body and the subject is instructed to point out exactly where he feels the touch. He is advised to report any other sensation (besides touch) which he might feel during the course of the test.
d. *Tactile discrimination:* It is the ability to distinguish between two adjacent touch stimuli. The subject is touched with two points of compass aesthesiometer, initially keeping the points close together and thereafter, separating them progressively. Each time the subject is asked whether he is being touched at one or two points. Tactile discrimination is greatest on finger tips and lips where even 1 to 2 mm of separation points can be recognised as two separate stimuli. However, on the back, the two points should be separated by atleast 30–70 mm to be distinguished as separate.

Position Sense

It is the ability to recognise the position of the joints and limbs in three dimensional spaces (proprioception).

The finger (or toe, ankle, knee, wrist or elbow) of the subject is moved up or down at the joints and he is asked to subsequently refer to that position. Normal people can recognise displacement of even a few degrees at all the joints.

Another way of doing this test is to hold one of the hands of the subject and move it in various directions through the air finally leaving it in some definite position. Now the subject is asked to put the other limb in a similar position.

Stereognosis

This sensation represents the ability to appreciate size, shape, weight, and form of the familiar objects by means of touch and pressure sensation without the help of vision.

The subject is asked to close his eyes and objects of the same shape but different sizes, e.g. matchsticks of different lengths are placed in his palm and he is asked to say which one is longer.

The subject is asked to name some familiar objects (e.g. coin, pencil and key, etc.) placed on his palm, keeping his eyes closed.

Vibration Sense

The foot of a low frequency (128 Hz) vibrating tuning fork is placed on some bony prominence in the region to be tested such as the shin of the tibia or the lateral malleolus or the dorsum of the finger. The subject is asked whether he feels the vibrations and also when he ceases to feel them. Then the examiner feels on himself.

Pain

- *Superficial pain:* The subject is pricked lightly with a sharp pin and inquired whether he feels the pain.
- *Deep pain:* The muscle of the subject is squeezed (arm muscles in upper limb and calf muscles and tendo-achilles in lower limb) and the subject is asked whether he feels the pain. Varying degrees of pain ranging from no pain to intense excessive pain may be felt.

Temperature

Two test tubes, one filled with warm and the other with cold water are used. The external surface of these test tubes is touched (one at a time) to the subject's part to be tested and he is asked to tell if he feels hot or cold.

Questions

1. Name the sensations lost with lesion in dorsal column.
2. Why tactile discrimination varies in different parts of the body?

EXPERIMENT NO. 8

AIM: TO RECORD VISUAL ACUITY OF THE SUBJECT

Definition

Visual acuity is the ability of the eye to recognise two point sources of light as separate.

It is expressed as minimum separable distance between two lines so that they can be perceived as separate.

Visual acuity is tested for distant vision and near vision

- For distant vision, Snellen's chart is used
- For near vision, Jaeger's chart is used.

Snellen's Chart

This chart is used for distant central visual acuity. The basis of this chart is the fact that two distant points can be visible as separate only when they subtend an angle of one minute at nodal point of the eye. The lines comprising the letter have such a breadth that they will subtend an angle of one minute at nodal point and each letter is so designed that it subtends an angle of five minutes at nodal point.

Testing for Distant Vision

Subject is seated comfortably at a distance of 6 m from the Snellen's chart. The illumination of the chart should not be less than 20 foot candles. Each eye is tested separately and one at a time. The subject is instructed to read the letters starting from top to the bottom line with the other eye covered.

Observation: According to the lines read, the visual acuity is expressed as 6/6 or 6/12 or 6/24 and so on, where denominator indicates the distance marked on the line which the subject is able to read comfortably and the numerator is the standard distance from which subject is asked to read the letters (6 meters normally). There are letters in different languages for different persons. For illiterates and children, letters C and E arranged in different position are used.

It top line is not read from 6 m distance, the subject is moved towards the chart in the increments of 1 m each time so as to read the top letter.

If top line is not read even from one meter distance then counting of fingers (CF) is done and vision is recorded as CF: 3m, CF: 2m or CF: 1 m.

If CF is absent then perception of hand movements (HM) is done so that vision is recorded as HM positive or negative.

If HM is also negative then light is thrown directly into the eye of the subject and he is asked whether he is able to perceive the light or not and the vision is recorded as PL (perception of light) positive or negative.

Testing for Near Vision

The Jaeger's chart is held by the subject at an ordinary reading distance and is asked to read the printed material of varying sizes down the chart. The print size ranges from N1–N5 with the largest print (N1) at the top and smallest (N5) at the bottom of the chart.

Observation: The near point is recorded as the smallest letter type which the subject can read comfortably.

Questions

1. What is near point and when does it recede?
2. Comment upon different refractory errors.

EXPERIMENT NO. 9

AIM: TO TEST COLOUR VISION

Colour vision is the function of cones. Different wavelengths of light are perceived as different colours by the retina.

Following tests are used for testing colour vision:

- Test using Ishihara's pseudoisochromatic colour plates
- Edridge green lantern test
- Holmgren's wool test.

Ishihara's Pseudoisochromatic Colour Plates (Fig. 5, Plate 3)

It is the most popular method for screening colour blindness in a population. These Ishihara's colour plates contain numbers in dots of primary colours painted on the background of dots of confusion colours in such a way that a colour blind person will not be able to read the number, or will read it as a different number from a normal person.

Edridge Green Lantern Test

It is a screening test employed to rule out colour blind persons for high risk jobs like drivers, pilots, etc. The Edridge green lantern contains glasses of various shades of colours fixed on the rotating discs which emit the light through an aperture. The intensity of the coloured beam can be varied simulating weather condition like fog, mist, rain, etc. through modified glasses like a ground glass to represent mist and a ribbed glass to represent fog of varying densities. The subject is asked to identify different colours shown to him.

Holmgren's Wool Test

This test consists of three different categories of coloured wool skeins:

- Test colour skeins
- Match colour skeins
- Confusion colour skeins.

The subject has to match the colour of the wool skein provided to him (test colour) from a heap of match colours and confusion colours. A normal person would pick up a similar wool skein, i.e. the match colour skein from the heap, but a colour blind person may pick up a skein of confusion colour.

Questions

1. Why it is necessary to perform the tests of colour vision?
2. Enumerate the abnormalities of colour vision.

EXPERIMENT NO. 10

AIM: TO PERFORM PERIMETRY

Perimetry is the process of plotting the field of vision or visual field of each eye.

Visual Field

Visual field is the sum of the images of the objects formed on the retina when the gaze is fixed at a particular point. Field of vision is limited by the size of the retina and margins of the orbit, nose and cheek.

Visual field extent with a test object of 5 mm diameter is

Temporal : 100°
Nasal : 60°
Superior : 60°
Inferior : 75°

Equipment

1. Perimeter
2. Perimeter chart
3. Test objects.

Perimeter

It consists of following parts:

- *Arc:* The perimeter arc is a metallic, calibrated, movable large arc of a circle with its concavity towards the subject, and graduations on convex surface from 0° to 90°, 0° being at the centre and the 90° at the periphery. The centre of the arc is occupied by a circular white spot which acts as a fixation point for fixing the gaze of the subject. It also bears a movable test object which is a white colour spot of 5 mm size.
- *Stand:* It provides stability to the perimeter on its vertical limbs. The arc is supported by a broad vertical limb.
- *Chin rest:* It is an adjustable rest and the subject's head is supported on it. It consists of two cups, of which left cup is used for testing right eye and vice versa.
- *Graduate dial:* Showing the meridians in which arc is adjusted.

Perimeter Chart

The central point of the chart corresponds with the visual axis and the concentric circles drawn around it are at 10° interval. Each concentric line denotes points of equal visual acuity called isopters. The radii of circles are marked at 15° intervals which denote different meridians. This chart rotates with the arc.

Test Object

Test objects of different sizes and colours can be used. Most commonly used test object is white in colour and 5 mm in diameter and is fixed to a holder in the arc.

Procedure

- The subject is asked to sit comfortably and the procedure is explained to him.

- In accordance with the eye to be tested, the subject's chin is placed on the chin rest appropriately (left chin rest for testing right eye and vice versa).
- The chart is mounted after positioning the arc in frontal plane on 0° meridian, in such a way that the 90° meridian on the chart should correspond with the arc and center of the chart should correspond with the visual axis.
- The spectacles, if used by the subject should be removed (if he can see comfortably without the spectacles) as the frame restricts the field of vision. However contact lens need not be removed. The subject is asked to cover the other eye with his hand and to fix the gaze of the test eye on the central fixation point.
- Starting from the temporal side of the eye to be tested, the test object is moved gradually from periphery towards the center till the subject perceives the object.
- The reading on the arc in degrees is noted and marked on the chart.
- Subsequent readings are taken at different meridians.
- Field of vision in obtained by joining these points. This constitutes monocular field of vision.
- The procedure is repeated for the other eye using appropriate chin rest.
- The field of vision can also be found using test objects of different sizes and colours.

Blind Spot

Physiological blind spot is the area in the field of vision where no image is formed. This area is devoid of rods and cones and is situated at the point where optic nerve leaves the eye ball. It lies about 15° laterals to the fixation point.

Mapping of Blind Spot

Blind spot can be mapped by keeping the arc in the horizontal meridian in the temporal quadrant. The whole test procedure is repeated. The object is continuously moved towards visual axis. The subject continues to see the object up to certain point and then the object disappears. The object reappears when moved further towards the fixation point. Both the points of disappearance and reappearance are marked and a circle is drawn which marks the blind spot. Another way to map the blind spot is by using "*Bjerrum screen*" and "*scotometer*".

Questions

1. How does pituitary adenoma affect the field of vision?
2. What do you understand by scotomas and how do you detect them?
3. What is binocular vision?

EXPERIMENT NO. 11

AIM: TO PERFORM HEARING TESTS

Following tests are commonly performed to assess the hearing of a subject:
1. Tuning fork tests
2. Audiometry.

Tuning Fork Tests

These tests are employed to test bone conduction and air conduction thereby differentiating conductive deafness from sensorineural deafness. A tuning fork of 512 Hz frequency is used. Three tests are commonly performed.

a. Rinne's test
b. Weber's test
c. Schwabach test.

Rinne's Test

i. A vibrating tuning fork is placed on the mastoid bone of the ear to be tested. The subject is asked to raise his hand when he stops hearing it.
ii. As soon as he stops hearing the vibration, the tuning fork is brought in front of his ear. He is asked whether the sound is audible or not.

Observation: If sound is heard in front of the external auditory canal, this means air conduction is better than bone conduction and Rinne's test is positive.

When bone conduction is better than air conduction, Rinne's test is designated as negative and is seen in conductive deafness.

In sensorineural deafness, air conduction is more than bone conduction as in a normal ear but in this case total duration of both air conduction and bone conduction is reduced.

Weber's Test

The base of the vibrating tuning fork is placed in the centre of the subject's forehead. The subject is asked whether the sound is heard equally in both the ears or it is louder on one side.

Observation: Normally Weber's test is centralised (i.e. heard by the subject equally in both ears)

- In conductive deafness—Sound is lateralised to diseased ear
- In sensorineural deafness—Sound is lateralised to normal ear.

Schwabach Test

In this test, bone conduction of the examiner and the subject is compared, considering the examiner to be normal. A vibrating tuning fork is placed on the subject's mastoid process and the subject is asked to raise his hand as soon as he stops hearing. Immediately the same tuning fork is now transferred to the mastoid process of the examiner.

Observation: The duration of hearing of the subject and the examiner should be equal i.e. the examiner should not be able to hear the sound after the subject has stopped hearing it.

- In sensorineural deafness the subject's bone conduction is lesser than that of the examiner.
- In conductive deafness, the subject's bone conduction is more than that of the examiner.

Audiometry

It is used for testing auditory acuity through quantitative assessment of hearing i.e. it tests the degree of deafness. In this test, the subject is presented with pure tones of various frequencies ranging from 250–8000 Hz (in a sound proof room with the help of sound attenuation headphones) and threshold intensity is determined at each frequency and plotted on a graph. One ear is tested at a time. This gives an objective assessment of the degree of deafness and the range of tones most affected. Bone conduction is also tested in a similar manner using a bone vibrating headset.

Questions

1. Why do we prefer tuning fork of frequency 512 Hz?
2. What do you understand by masking of sound?
3. Why bone conduction is more than air conduction in diseases affecting middle ear?

EXPERIMENT NO. 12

AIM: TO DETERMINE VISUAL AND AUDITORY REACTION TIME

Introduction

Reaction time refers to the time taken by an individual to respond to a stimulus. However, reaction is different from a reflex as the former is a voluntary action in response to a consciously perceived stimulus. Visual reaction time is the time taken to react to a visual stimulus (lighted bulb) and auditory reaction time denotes time required to react to an auditory stimulus (sound of tapping of the tapping key).

Equipment

Kymograph, electromagnetic signal marker, low voltage terminal/AC time clock, tapping keys, bulb.

Visual Reaction Time

Procedure

- Two tapping keys (key I and key II), a bulb placed in between two keys and a signal marker are connected in series to a low voltage terminal (AC time clock if low voltage terminal is not available).
- The recording of the movement of signal marker is done on kymograph moving at the speed of 560 mm/second.
- The subject is asked to gently press the key II and instructed to release the key as soon as he observes the lighted bulb.
- The examiner presses the key I and bulb is lighted.
- The time elapsed between lighting of the bulb and release of the key II by the subject is recorded as a deflection of the signal marker on the kymograph and is known as visual reaction time.
- Normal visual reaction time is 150–225 milliseconds.

Auditory Reaction Time

Procedure

- Setup is same as above except that bulb is not included in the circuit and the tapping sound of the tapping key acts as an auditory stimulus for the subject.
- The subject is asked to gently press the key II and instructed to release the key as soon as he hears the sound of tapping of the key by the examiner.
- The examiner presses the key I in such a manner that the tapping makes a sound.
- The time elapsed between hearing of the tapping sound and release of the key II by the subject is recorded as a deflection of the signal marker on the kymograph and is known as auditory reaction time.
- Normal auditory reaction time is 120–185 milliseconds.

Questions

1. Why visual reaction time is longer than auditory reaction time?
2. Name the factors affecting reaction time.

AIM: TO DETERMINE VISUAL AND AUDITORY REACTION TIME

Introduction

[illegible]

Equipment

[illegible]

Visual Reaction Time

DEMONSTRATION NO. 1

AIM: TO RECORD EEG USING DATA ACQUISITION AND ANALYSIS SYSTEM

The electroencephalogram (EEG) is the graphical representation of electrical activity of various areas of brain obtained due to rhythmic discharge of neuronal cell bodies in the superficial layers of cortical grey matter. It forms an important diagnostic tool for epilepsy, organic brain diseases and head injury.

Equipment

Different instruments are available to obtain EEG with a basic set up as follows:
- Data acquisition and analysis system (Fig. 6, Plate 3)
- EEG electrode—Disc/cup electrodes to be placed on the scalp
- EEG recording gel/paste—To reduce the resistance between electrodes and scalp.

Procedure

- EEG parameters are set using software of the equipment.
- The EEG electrodes are placed on the subject's scalp with the subject in sitting/lying down position comfortably taking care that the scalp is not oily.
- Electrodes are prepositioned as per the international 10–20 montage system in which electrodes are placed in reference to following important bony landmarks.
  - Nasion: The point of indentation between nose and forehead
  - Inion: The junction between back of head and neck just at the occipital protuberance
  - Pre-auricular points: Near the tragus.
- Leads from the electrodes terminate in 2 mm pin plugs which in turn are connected to input on the console.
- EEG recording is done using two channels at a time.
- Baseline tracing is recorded.
- Recording is done for various wave forms like alpha, beta, delta and theta activity.

EEG Rhythm	Frequency (Hz)	Amplitude (μV)	Prominent area of occurrence
Alpha (α)	8–13	30–70	Parietal, occipital
Beta (β)	14–30	5–10	Parietal, frontal
Theta (θ)	4–7	50–100	Parietal and temporal
Delta (δ)	1–4	20–200	Cortex independent of subcortical regions of brain

- Different tracings are taken to see the effect of the following:
  - Eyes closed and mind relaxed
  - Eyes opened
  - Mathematical calculation
  - Photic stimulation
  - Hyperventilation.

Analysis of EEG

- Analysis and interpretation of EEG waveform is done in terms of amplitude, frequency and predominant wave types obtained in various leads.

- FFT analysis is done after selecting the time periods of activity.
- Power spectrum analysis of acquired EEG signal is also done.

Questions

1. Name the clinical conditions in which abnormal EEG wave forms are obtained?
2. What do you understand by alpha block?

DEMONSTRATION NO. 2

AIM: TO RECORD GALVANIC SKIN RESPONSE USING DATA ACQUISITION AND ANALYSIS SYSTEM

Introduction

It is the record of electrical potentials from the skin surface in response to stimuli causing sympathetic activation. It is also known as sympathetic skin response. Sweat glands of the skin are innervated by sympathetic nervous system. When sympathetic activity increases (arousal), the sweat gland secretion increases and the skin conductivity for electrical potentials increases.

Equipments

- Data acquisition and analysis system
- Electrodermal activity amplifier
- Electrodermal activity electrodes
- Electrode gel.

Procedure

- Setting of GSR parameters is done by using the software of the instrument in use.
- After proper cleaning of the skin, the active electrode is placed on the palm (or sole of the foot), the reference electrode on the dorsum of hand (or foot) and the ground in between the two.
- The subject is seated in a calm environment and is made to relax.
- Baseline tracing is recorded by applying a constant current of 5 microamperes and response is noted in terms of latency and amplitude.
- The subject is distracted by giving a sudden stimulus like clapping and the response is observed.
- Abnormal GSR is observed in progressive autonomic dysfunction.

Questions

1. How is the galvanic skin response related to changes in skin conductance?

DEMONSTRATION NO. 3

AIM: TO RECORD VISUAL EVOKED POTENTIALS (VEP) USING DATA ACQUISITION AND ANALYSIS SYSTEM

Introduction

Visual evoked potentials are the changes in electrical potentials recorded from the scalp in response to visual stimuli. They represent the response of cortical and subcortical structures to photic stimulation. Recording of VEPs helps in ascertaining the intactness of visual pathways.

Equipment

- Data acquisition and analysis system
- Disc type EEG electrodes
- Electrode gel/paste
- LED goggles/black and white checker board.

Procedure

- The subject is instructed to stop using any miotic or mydriatic agent at least 12 hours before the test.
- The subject is advised not to use hair spray or hair oil after hair wash before the test.
- Parameters are set as per the software of the equipment.
- The subject is seated in a calm environment and is asked to be relaxed.
- After proper cleaning of the skin at the points of placement of electrodes, the active electrode is placed at Oz (occipital region), the reference electrode at Fpz, i.e. 12 cm above the nasion. Linked ear reference electrode can also be used in addition. The ground electrode is placed at Cz, i.e. vertex.
- The subject is asked to wear LED goggles or he is asked to fix the gaze in the centre of the computer screen and visual stimuli are delivered.
- One eye is tested at a time.
- The recording parameters are set as follows:
  - Low cut filter—1–3 Hz
  - High cut filter—100–300 Hz
  - Sensitivity—2μV/div
  - Sweep speed—50–100 msec/div
  - Number of epochs averaged—200
  - Electrode impedence—<5 kohms.
- Record of various wave forms, i.e. N_{75}, P_{100} and N_{135} is obtained and their peak latency and peak-to-peak amplitude is measured and analysed. N denotes negative and P denotes positive waveform while number subscript depicts time taken (msec) to obtain the particular waveform after stimulation.
- Most commonly used parameter for analysis in VEP is peak latency, duration and amplitude of the wave form P_{100}.
- The latency of P_{100} is increased in demyelinating disorders of optic pathways like in *optic neuritis*, *glaucoma* and *multiple sclerosis*.

- Optic nerve compression can cause both increase in latency and decrease in amplitude of P_{100}, like in severe *papilloedema* and *pituitary tumour*.

Questions

1. What do you understand by the term VEP? Mention its significance.
2. What are the prerequisites for recording of VEP?

DEMONSTRATION NO. 4

AIM: TO RECORD BRAINSTEM AUDITORY EVOKED POTENTIALS (BAEP) USING DATA ACQUISITION AND ANALYSIS SYSTEM

Introduction

These are the changes in electrical potentials generated by sequential activation of different parts of auditory pathway, recorded from the ear and vertex in response to brief auditory stimulation. The procedure is also named as *brainstem evoked response audiometry (BERA)*. Recording of BAEP helps in assessing the conduction in the auditory pathway and degree of hearing deficit. It is particularly useful in infants and young children suspected of being deaf.

Equipment

- Data acquisition and analysis system
- Disc type EEG electrodes
- Electrode gel/paste
- Headphones for auditory stimulus.

Procedure

- The subject is advised not to use hair spray or hair oil after hair wash before the test.
- Parameters are set as per the software of the equipment.
- The subject is seated in a calm environment and is made to relax.
- After proper cleaning of the skin at the points of placement of electrodes, the active electrodes are placed on both the ear lobes or mastoid processes, the reference electrode is placed at vertex and the ground electrode is placed at Fz.
- The subject is asked to wear shielded headphones and auditory stimulus in the form of auditory click (a square wave pulse of 0.1 msec duration) is delivered.
- One ear is tested at a time.
- The recording parameters are set as follows:
  - Low cut filter—10–100 Hz
  - High cut filter—3000 Hz
  - Sensitivity—0.5μV/div
  - Sweep speed—1 msec/ div
  - Number of epochs averaged—2000
  - Electrode impedance—<5 k-ohms
  - Stimulus intensity—70dB
- Record of various wave forms wave, i.e. from wave I to wave V is obtained that depicts the following:
  - Wave I—From peripheral part of cochlear nerve
  - Wave II—From cochlear nuclei
  - Wave III—From superior olivary nucleus

- Wave IV—From lateral leminiscus
- Wave V—From inferior colliculus.

- Wave VI and VII are sometimes observed which represent activity of medial geniculate body and auditory radiation respectively.
- Analysis of BAEP is done by calculating absolute latencies of waves I to V, absolute amplitude of all waves, different interpeak latencies, i.e. wave I–III, III–V and I–V and amplitude ratio of wave V/I.
- Interpeak latency I–III is a measure of conduction from VIIIth nerve across sub-arachnoid space into lower pons; III–V interpeak latency is a measure of conduction from lower pons to midbrain. Interpeak latency I–V is commonly used clinical entity representing conduction from proximal cochlear nerve through pons to mid-brain.
- Absence of a wave form indicates lesion in the area represented by that wave.
- Interpeak latencies get prolonged in *demyelination, ischaemia* and *tumours*.

Questions

1. Draw and label various wave forms of BAEP.
2. What are the factors affecting BAEP?

DEMONSTRATION NO. 5

AIM: TO PERFORM AUTONOMIC FUNCTION TESTS

The autonomic nervous system comprises of postganglionic sympathetic and parasympathetic neurons in the periphery and their preganglionic components in the intermediolateral cell columns of the spinal cord and their rostral connections in the brainstem. The following autonomic function tests are commonly performed:

Deep Breath Test

It is a test of parasympathetic influence on cardiovascular system. The patient is asked to lie supine comfortably. When the pulse is steady, the subject is asked to take deep breaths at a rate of about six breaths per minute for one minute, i.e. six maximal deep breaths. The difference between the maximal and the minimal heart rates is observed.

Interpretation: Normally there is a difference of more than 15 beats per minute between maximum and minimum heart rates. However, in autonomic disturbances, this difference is less than 10 beats per minute.

Another expression of this test is *E:I ratio*, i.e. the ratio of longest R-R interval (maximum slowing of heart during expiration) to the shortest R-R interval (maximum increase in heart rate during inspiration) obtained in the same ECG recording.

Interpretation: Ratio of more than 1.06 is considered as normal.

Valsalva Test

This test is done for assessment of parasympathetic function. Valsalva manoeuvre consists of a brief period of forced expiration against closed glottis. The patient, while in sitting posture, blows into a sphygmomanometer, maintaining a pressure of 40 mmHg for 15 seconds while a continuous ECG is recorded. The ratio of longest R-R interval after the manoeuvre to the shortest R-R interval during the manoeuvre gives the Valsalva ratio.

Interpretation: A Valsalva ratio of ≥ 1.21 is considered as normal, while a ratio of 1.11–1.20 as borderline and the ratio of 1.1 or less indicates autonomic dysfunction.

Isometric Exercise

It is also known as *Handgrip test* and is done to assess sympathetic function. Baseline blood pressure recordings (systolic as well as diastolic) are taken. Using the hand dynamometer, the subject is asked to perform *Maximal voluntary contraction* (MVC) as long as possible. The maximum force exerted is noted down. After giving rest for some time, the subject is made to perform isometric exercise at 30% of maximal voluntary contraction for 5 minutes. Blood pressure is recorded every minute during the period of exercise. The response to the test is taken as the difference between the mean of 3 resting diastolic blood pressure recordings and the last reading of blood pressure during exercise (i.e. just before the release of handgrip). *Interpretation:* An increase in diastolic blood pressure by more than 16 mmHg is taken as normal, an increase by 11–15 mmHg as borderline and increase in diastolic blood pressure by less than 10 mmHg indicates autonomic dysfunction.

Change of Posture

a. *Heart rate response to change in posture (30:15 ratio)*: The subject is made to lie down quietly for 2 minutes. Resting blood pressure and ECG are recorded. The subject is asked to standup unaided from lying down position quickly and remain standing for about one minute. The longest R-R interval in ECG (which denotes slowest heart rate and occurs at around 30th beat after standing) divided by shortest R-R interval (fastest heart rate occurring at around 15th beat after standing) gives 30:15 ratio and is used as an index for vagal function and hence parasympathetic activity.

   Interpretation: Normal ratio is more than 1.03. A ratio of less than 1 is considered abnormal.

b. *Blood pressure response to change in posture:* After taking the resting blood pressure and pulse rate in lying down position, the subject is asked to stand up unaided and quickly. The blood pressure and the pulse rate are recorded, 2 minutes after standing.

   Interpretation: A sustained drop in systolic BP by more than 20mmHg or diastolic by more than 10 mmHg after standing for at least 2 minutes that is not associated with an increase in pulse rate of more than 15 beats per minute suggests an autonomic deficit and differentiates autonomic failure from sluggish baroreceptor responses that are common in old age. In non-neurogenic causes of orthostatic hypotension, the blood pressure fall is accompanied by increase in heart rate by more than 15 beats per min.

c. *Head-up tilt:* The person is asked to take rest in supine position for at least 20 minutes before starting the test. Passive tilting of the subject through 80 degrees from recumbent towards the erect position is done using a tilt table while serial recording of blood pressure is done.

   Interpretation: In normal subjects, passive tilting causes a small decrease in systolic blood pressure and increase in diastolic blood pressure and heart rate but in patients with unexplained syncope or vagally mediated syncope, tilt produces symptomatic hypotension and syncope within 10–30 minutes.

Cold Pressor Test

This test assesses sympathetic function and is an index of vasoconstrictor tone. Baseline blood pressure is recorded. One hand of the subject is immersed up to the wrist in the cold water at 4°C temperature for 1 minute. Blood pressure is recorded at 30 seconds and 1 minute of submersion of the hand in cold water and after taking out the hand, every minute, till the value returns to baseline.

Interpretation: In normal subjects, there is an increase in systolic and diastolic blood pressure by at least 10–20 mmHg. An increase of less than 10 mmHg indicates autonomic dysfunction. An increase of more than 20/20 mmHg indicates vascular hyper-reactivity which can be observed in hypertensive patients and in persons at a risk of developing hypertension later in life.

Questions

1. Explain the heart rate and blood pressure changes during Valsalva manoeuvre.
2. Explain the basis of cold pressor response.

DEMONSTRATION NO. 6

AIM: TO PERFORM OPHTHALMOSCOPY

Ophthalmoscopy is the examination of the fundus of the eye ball, which includes retina, optic disc, choroid and blood vessels, with the help of an ophthalmoscope.

It is done as a part of the eye examination to:

a. Detect problems or diseases of the eye, e.g. glaucoma, retinal detachment, optic neuritis, etc.
b. Help diagnose other conditions or diseases that may affect the eye secondarily, e.g. diabetes, hypertension, etc. which may present as papilloedema or other manifestations in retina.

Ophthalmoscopy can be performed by three methods:

- Distant direct ophthalmoscopy
- Direct ophthalmoscopy
- Indirect ophthalmoscopy.

Distant Direct Ophthalmoscopy

The subject is asked to sit in a dark room and light is thrown into his eye from a distance of 20–25 cm. The examiner first sees a reddish reflex coming through the pupil. This shows that lens is transparent and that light is shining all the way through the fluid filled eye ball to the back of the eye and on to the retina. This examination is useful in diagnosing any opacity in refractive media which is seen as a black shadow in a red glow.

Direct Ophthalmoscopy

It is the most common type of ophthalmoscopic examination performed in clinics.

Principle

A convergent beam of light is focused into the pupil of the subject. The parallel rays emerging from the subject's eyes are brought to focus on the retina of the emmetropic observer through the viewing hole in the ophthalmoscope. The image formed in this case is erect, virtual and about 15 times magnified.

Procedure

The subject is seated in a dark room and is asked to look straight ahead at some distant point. The clinician sits/stands by the side of the subject's eye to be examined. Right eye of the subject is examined with the right eye of the clinician and vice versa. The clinician looks through the ophthalmoscope and moves along with it, very close to the face of the subject and bright light is shone into his eye. The subject is asked to hold the eyes steady without blinking. As the retina is focused the details are examined systematically starting from optic disc, blood vessels, the four quadrants of general background and macula.

Indirect Ophthalmoscopy

It gives a better and wider view of the retina than direct ophthalmoscopy. It is generally done with a binocular ophthalmoscope with head band or that mounted on a spectacle frame. It is done after instilling eye drops which dilate the pupil. This examination takes 5–10 minutes and needs more expertise.

Principle

The principle is to make the eye highly myopic by placing a strong convex lens in front of patients' eye so that emergent rays from retina are brought to focus between lens and the observer's eye as real, inverted and magnified image.

Procedure

The subject is asked to sit in reclining position in a dark room. The eyes of the subject are held open by the examiner. Light is shone into the eye and examination is done through a special condensing lens (+20 D routinely) first placed closed to the subject's eye and then slowly moved towards the examiner until the image of the retina is clearly seen. The subject is asked to look into different directions to examine different quadrants of fundus.

Features of following structures of retina are usually observed with the ophthalmoscope:

1. *Vessels:* These are the small arteries and veins that supply blood to retina. Veins appear darker and larger than arteries by a ratio of 3:2 and sometimes also seen to be pulsating. If arteries are much smaller than this, it may indicate *premature damage of arteries (arteriosclerosis).*
2. *Optic disc and cup:* Optic nerve enters into the eye ball at this place. It is considered as physiological blind spot. Optic disc appears as a circle of reddish brown colour while the cup is a smaller circle inside the disc which is more yellowish and pink in colour. These are located at the centre of the retina at the back of the eye. The cup is the head of the optic nerve. Normally cup and disc are round with distinct margins or edges. The diameter of the cup should be equal to or less than 1/3rd of the diameter of the disc. Enlarged cup indicates *glaucoma.*
3. *Surface of retina:* It is reddish brown in colour with blood vessels spread over it like a cob web. Vessels with leakage of fluid and blood indicate abnormal pattern.
4. *Macula:* It is the area of the retina near the posterior pole of the eye which has highest visual acuity. To look at the macula, the subject has to look directly into the light coming from the ophthalmoscope. It is dusky in appearance and has no vessels crossing it.

Question

1. Mention the clinical significance of ophthalmoscopy.

Chapter 4

Nerve Muscle Physiology Experiments

EXPERIMENT NO. 1

AIM: TO STUDY THE PHENOMENON OF FATIGUE USING MOSSO'S ERGOGRAPH

Introduction

Phenomenon of fatigue is observed by voluntary and isotonic contraction of the middle finger up to the point of fatigue, after being subjected to varying loads, frequencies, venous and arterial occlusion.

Equipment

Ergograph with weights, sphygmomanometer, metronome or seconds watch.

Equipment Description

Ergograph consists of a wooden platform with clamps for holding the forearm and two metallic tubes to fix the index finger and ring finger. A pulley is fixed on one side of the wooden platform, over which a string is passed to hang the weights. A loop is made on the other side of the string to hold the middle finger for pulling the weights. A spring loaded writing device is present on one side of the wooden platform with a pen/pencil holder and space for fixing the paper for recording the excursions. The arrangement of writing device is such that after recording of each excursion, the writing device moves ahead automatically. Another method of recording the excursions is on a kymograph through a lever system.

Procedure

- A pencil/writing pen and the paper is fixed in the writing device.
- Forearm of the dominant hand is fixed on the wooden board with the help of clamps.
- A fixed weight (2 kg) is hung on the string.
- Middle finger (second phalange) is placed in the loop of the string.
- Metronome is switched on and its frequency is fixed at 30/minute.

- With the help of middle finger, weights are pulled and released at a fixed frequency corresponding to the click of the metronome, up to the point of fatigue, i.e. till the subject is no longer able to contract his finger.
- Simultaneous recording is obtained as each pull of the finger marks the excursion on the paper at 2 kg, 30/minute values.
- Considering this weight and frequency as control, the effect of increasing the weight (3 Kg) while keeping the frequency constant and then increasing the frequency (60/min) while keeping the weight constant is recorded.
- The effect of venous occlusion is obtained by inflating the sphygmomanometer cuff tied around the arm and maintaining the cuff pressure at 40 mmHg. The experiment is performed with 2 Kg weight and frequency of 30 per minute.
- The effect of arterial occlusion on the onset of fatigue can be obtained by inflating the sphygmomanometer cuff up to 160–170 mmHg, maintained at this level and experiment is repeated with the control values, taking care to deflate the cuff immediately after the subject stops performing the test.
- Work done (W) is calculated in each case by following formula.

  W = force (weight in gm) × distance (total length of recording obtained in cm) × 981 ergs.
- The results obtained are compared and interpreted.

Questions

1. Comment on the first seat of fatigue in human beings and in isolated nerve muscle preparation.
2. How does venous occlusion affect the isotonic exercise?

DEMONSTRATION NO. 1

AIM: TO RECORD EMG USING DATA ACQUISITION AND ANALYSIS SYSTEM

Electromyography (EMG) is the record of electrical potentials in a muscle during its contraction. Resting muscle does not show any spontaneous electrical activity due to minimal and asynchronous discharge from motor units.

Equipment

- Data acquisition and analysis system
- Adhesive/disposable surface electrodes/needle electrodes
- One unshielded electrode for ground.

Procedure

- EMG parameters are set as per the software of the equipment.
- To measure the EMG activity from a muscle, the two shielded electrodes are placed on two separate points on that muscle.
- The active electrode is placed at the point of maximum activity of that muscle and reference electrode at a small distance from the first one.
- One unshielded electrode is placed on the forearm for grounding.
- The electrodes are connected through a pre amplifier to the recording system.
- Normal baseline tracing is taken.
- Recording is done with graded levels of muscle activity with a hand dynamometer and during muscle relaxation.
- For performing the needle EMG, a needle electrode is inserted in the belly of the concerned muscle and insertional activity, spontaneous activity and voluntary activity is recorded in sequence:
  - Insertional activity is the brief burst of electrical activity for 5–10 msec, due to needle insertion. It is increased in *denervated muscle* and decreased in *myopathies*.
  - Spontaneous activity is absent in a normal muscle except miniature end plate potential observed if the needle is near the end plate region (monophasic negative waves). Abnormal spontaneous activity includes fibrillations, fasciculations and cramps.
  - Voluntary contractions in which person is asked to increase contraction of the said muscle. With increased contractions, more and more MUP's run into each other called interference pattern.
- Motor unit potentials (MUPs) are recorded and analysed for their frequency, duration, amplitude, phases and rise time:
  - Motor unit potentials represent the sum of action potentials of muscle fibres supplied by a motor neuron (motor unit).
  - Frequency of firing of MUP is 5–15 Hz during mild contraction which increases with recruitment of motor units during voluntary activity.
  - Duration of normal MUP is taken as the time taken from the initial take off of the MUP to the point of return to the base line. Normal duration is 5–10 msec. Duration of MUP is increased in lower

motor neuron disease and neuropathies. Short duration MUP is observed in children, myopathies and myasthenia gravis.

- Amplitude of MUP is from peak of positive deflection to the peak of negative deflection. Normal value is 0.5–2 mV. It is a measure of size, density and type of muscle fibre.
- Phases of MUP as recorded by needle EMG are triphasic, i.e. positive, negative, positive deflection. MUP's with more than 4 phases are called as polyphasic potentials and are observed in myopathies during regeneration of fibres.
- Rise time of MUP is the time duration from initial positive to the next negative peak. Normal value is around 500 μsec. It indicates the distance of needle electrode from the muscle fibre.

EMG can also be recorded on Physiograph.

Recording on Physiograph

Equipment

- Physiograph/polyrite
- 3 Surface electrodes
- Biopotential coupler
- Paper roll.

Procedure

- Coupler is plugged into the console with the console mains off.
- Physiograph is calibrated.
- Mode is set at EMG.
- 50 Hz filter is put on.
- Two surface electrodes are placed at two points on a muscle whose activity is to be recorded.
- One surface electrode is placed on the wrist which is the ground electrode.
- Electrodes from the subject are connected to three pin junction box and the junction box to the coupler.
- Paper is run using thumb screw on the console.
- Baseline tracing is taken with the muscle relaxed.
- Subject is asked to contract the muscle and recording is taken.

Observation

- Relaxed healthy muscle shows no electrical activity.
- As the muscle starts contracting and as the muscular activity increases, more motor units are recruited which is seen as deflection on the paper.

Questions

1. What do you understand by recruitment of motor units?
2. What are the different types of abnormal spontaneous activity?
3. Draw and label a normal motor unit potential.

DEMONSTRATION NO. 2

AIM: TO RECORD NERVE CONDUCTION VELOCITY USING DATA ACQUISITION AND ANALYSIS SYSTEM

Determination of nerve conduction velocity is an important electrodiagnostic tool in neurological testing to assess the functional status of peripheral nerves. Motor and sensory nerve conduction velocity (MNCV and SNCV) are usually determined. Various peripheral motor nerves commonly studied are median nerve, ulnar nerve and radial nerve (upper limb) and sciatic nerve, posterior tibial nerve and common peroneal nerve (lower limb). SNCV is generally determined for ulnar and median nerve in upper limb and superficial peroneal and sural nerve in lower limb.

Equipments

- Data acquisition and analysis system
- Nerve stimulator
- EMG/EP electrode box
- EMG surface electrodes
- Ground electrode
- Electrode jelly/paste.

Procedure

- Hardware is set up.
- Two surface electrodes, i.e. the active electrode and reference electrode are placed over the muscle belly at motor point and near the tendon of the muscle respectively, supplied by the nerve under study. Ground electrode is placed at a short distance away.
- All these surface and ground electrodes are connected to the EMG/EP electrode box.
- Stimulating electrodes are placed lengthwise along the nerve to be stimulated taking care that the positive end of the stimulator and the surface electrodes should approximate each other.
- The stimulation is given first at the distal end of the nerve and then at the proximal end of the nerve, each time starting with a lower voltage and subsequently increasing until the required threshold is reached and the waveform obtained.
- Waveform is analyzed and conduction time is noted.
- Distance is measured from stimulating to recording electrodes with the help of a measuring tape.

Analysis and Calculation

- The attributes of motor nerve conduction that are measured are as follows:
  - Onset latency of *Compound muscle action potential* (CMAP) is the time from appearance of stimulus artifact to the first negative deflection of CMAP. It denotes time taken for neuromuscular transmission and that for propagation of impulse along the muscle membrane. Increase in latency indicates *"demyelination"*.
  - Amplitude of CMAP is measured from base line to negative peak (base to peak) or between negative and positive peaks (peak to peak). Decrease in amplitude suggests axonal loss in nerve fibre.

- Duration of CMAP is measured from onset to negative peak, or to the positive peak or up to the final return of wave form to the base line and it depicts density of small fibres.

- Nerve conduction velocity is determined after calculating the difference in latent periods of wave forms of compound muscle action potential (CMAP) obtained at two stimulation sites and dividing it with the distance between stimulating and recording electrode.

Nerve conduction velocity in the nerve = D/time, in m/sec

- Sensory nerve conduction is measured in the same manner with same attributes as motor nerve. However sensory nerve action potential can be measured by two methods, i.e. measurement of *orthodromic conduction* or *antidromic conduction*. Both types of measurements provide same kind of information.
- For orthodromic conduction measurement, stimulation is done at distal part of nerve and recording is done at a proximal point of the nerve. Ring electrodes are used for stimulation.
- For antidromic conduction measurement, stimulation is done at proximal part of nerve and recording is done at a distal point of the nerve. Surface electrodes are used for stimulation.
- Motor nerve conduction velocity in median nerve is around 54–62 m/sec and sensory nerve conduction velocity in median nerve is 40–50/sec.
- Sites of surface electrode placement and sites of stimulation of nerves are tabulated below

Name of nerve	Recording electrode	Stimulation site I (SI)	Stimulation site II (SII)	Stimulation site III (SIII)	Stimulation site IV (S IV)
		MNCV			
Median nerve	Abductor pollicis brevis	Wrist	Elbow	Axilla	Erb's point
Ulnar nerve	Abductor digiti minimi	Wrist	Elbow	Axilla	Erb's point
Radial nerve	Abductor pollicis longus	Elbow	Triceps	Axilla	Erb's point
Common paroneal nerve	Extensor digitorum brevis	Ankle (anterior)	Head of fibula		
Tibial nerve	Abductor hallucis	Medial malleolus	Popliteal fossa		
Sciatic nerve	Paroneal innervated—Extensor digitorum brevis Tibial innervated—Abductor hallucis	Gluteal fold	Apex of popliteal fossa for medial trunk	Head of fibula for lateral trunk	
		SNCV			
Median nerve	Ring electrodes at interphalangeal joints of index finger	Wrist			
Ulnar nerve	Ring electrodes at interphalangeal joints of little finger	Wrist			
Radial nerve	First web space	10–15 cm proximal to recording electrode at lateral edge of radius			
superficial peroneal nerve	Just above the junction of lateral third of the line joining malleoli anteriorly	10–15 cm proximal to upper edge of lateral malleolus anteriorly	Head of fibula		
Sural nerve	Between lateral malleolus and tendo Achilles	10–15 cm proximal to recording electrode distal to lower border of gastrocnemius posteriorly			

Questions

1. What are the factors affecting nerve conduction velocity?
2. What is the clinical significance of determining nerve conduction velocity?
3. Write down various types of classification of nerve fibres.

Chapter

5

Reproductive System

DEMONSTRATION

AIM: TO PERFORM PREGNANCY TEST

Following three types of tests are performed for detection of pregnancy:

1. Immunological tests
2. Biological tests
3. Radioimmunoassay.

The immunological tests are most commonly used in laboratory.

Principle

This test is based on antigen (β-hCG in urine sample of pregnant female) and antibody (anti-hCG antibody/antisera) reaction. If the urine sample contains hCG it will neutralize the anti-hCG antibody and hence will not allow agglutination with hCG antigen coated on latex particles. However, if hCG is absent in urine sample the free anti-hCG antibody will react with the hCG antigen and results in agglutination. Thus agglutination in the sample indicates negative pregnancy test and vice versa. This principle is known as latex agglutination inhibition assay.

Material Provided in the Kit

- hCG antibody/antisera
- Latex particles coated with β-hCG antigen
- Reusable glass slide
- Disposable mixing sticks
- Disposable dropper.

Procedure

- The first morning sample of urine (test sample) of the patient is taken.

- One drop of urine of the test sample is put on one side of the slide and one drop of urine of a non-pregnant female (control) on the other side of the slide.
- One drop of antiserum is added on each side and the sample is mixed on each side with separate sticks.
- One drop of β-hCG antigen is added on both sides. The contents are mixed for about two minutes. The results are interpreted.

Result

- If agglutination is present within two minutes—Pregnancy test negative.
- If agglutination is absent within two minutes—Pregnancy test positive.

Questions

1. Name the most sensitive test in terms of time frame for detection of pregnancy.
2. Name the biological tests for pregnancy.
3. Name the hormones secreted by placenta during pregnancy.

Chapter 6

Mammalian Experiments

DEMONSTRATION NO. 1

AIM: TO RECORD BLOOD PRESSURE AND RESPIRATION IN MAMMALIAN (RABBIT) PREPARATION AND TO STUDY THE EFFECT OF (A) CAROTID OCCLUSION (B) VAGUS STIMULATION AND (C) DRUGS

Equipments

Polyrite, Pressure transducer, Arterial cannula, Tracheostomy tube, Student stimulator, 3-way adaptor, various Drugs

Procedure

1. *Anaesthesia:* Rabbit is made to fast overnight. The dose for anaesthetic agent (urethane) is calculated as per weight of the rabbit. Urethane (0.5–1.5 g/kg body weight) is injected intravenously through pinna vein. As the rabbit is completely anaesthetised, the respiration becomes deep and regular, voluntary movements and corneal reflex disappear.
2. The rabbit is placed supine and the limbs are tied onto the operating table. The skin is shaved over the trachea and the inguinal region.
3. *Dissection of trachea:* Trachea is dissected out by giving a midline vertical incision on the ventral surface of neck, cutting through the skin and subcutaneous tissue and retracting the overlying muscles. Once the trachea is exposed, a transverse incision is given over the 2nd or 3rd tracheal ring. A tracheal cannula is inserted into the trachea and a tight ligature is applied to keep it in position. The free end of tracheal cannula is attached to the thermistor transducer, which in turn is connected to one channel of polyrite to record the respiratory excursions.
4. *Dissection of femoral artery:* The femoral artery is palpated in the inguinal region. A long vertical incision is given parallel to the location of the artery starting from the mid-inguinal point. The skin, subcutaneous tissue and deep tissue are separated by gentle dissection with an artery forceps. The femoral vessels and nerve lie beneath this. Femoral artery is cleared of the tissues and a ligature is made at the lower end of the visualised part of the artery. An arterial cannula is inserted into the artery after

giving a fine nick in the artery. It is kept in position with help of a tight ligature. The other end of the cannula is attached to a pressure transducer filled with heparinised saline which in turn is connected to another channel of polyrite to record the blood pressure tracings.

5. *Dissection of vagus nerve and carotid artery:* Vagus nerve and carotid artery lie along both sides of trachea in the carotid sheath in the neck. The carotid artery is palpated and dissected out. Thread is passed separately around carotid artery and vagus nerve.

Recording (Figs 6.1 to 6.5)

1. *Calibration of the polyrite:* Calibration of the polyrite is done prior to recording of the blood pressure. The arterial cannula with three way adaptor is attached to a pressure transducer which in turn is connected to the designated channel of the polyrite for measuring blood pressure. The second limb of the three way adaptor is connected to the mercury manometer and the third limb of the adaptor is attached to a 10 ml syringe filled with heparinised saline. The polyrite is balanced by using the coarse and fine balance voltage keeping the pen position in center. Once it is balanced, the pen is brought at the lower most point. The pressure inside the transducer is increased by pressing the plunger of the syringe in a graded manner. Simultaneous increase in pressure in the manometer and the corresponding pen deflection on the polyrite at that particular pressure is marked on the paper of the polyrite.
2. Recording of normal blood pressure and respiration is done on the moving paper of the polyrite and the effect of following variables on blood pressure and respiration is recorded.
   i. *Carotid occlusion*:
      a. The common carotid artery on one side is occluded for few seconds, with the help of a bulldog clamp and the effect over blood pressure and respiration is recorded.
      b. The effect of occlusion of the carotid artery above the carotid sinus and the electrical stimulation of the carotid sinus can also be recorded.

   ii. *Vagus nerve stimulation*:
      a. The vagus nerve on one side is stimulated electrically at varying strength and frequency of stimulation and the effect over blood pressure and respiration is recorded each time.
      b. The effect of stimulation of peripheral cut end and central cut end of vagus after cutting the vagus nerve can also be recorded.

   iii. *Effect of drugs*:
      The effect of following drugs is recorded
      a. *Adrenaline*: In a dose of 3 μg/kg body weight (Intravenous)
      b. *Acetylcholine*: In a dose of 10 μg/kg body weight (Intravenous)
      c. *Atropine sulphate*: In a dose of 2 mg/kg body weight (Intravenous).

   The dose response curve is obtained with a graded increase in the dosage of the drug.

Precautions

1. The effect of one drug is properly washed off before looking for the effect of the other drug.
2. Stimulatory drugs are always given first.

Questions

1. Define *Traube-Hering* and *Mayer* waves. Give their physiological significance.
2. Explain the effect of vagus nerve stimulation on heart rate and blood pressure. What is post-vagal potentiation?

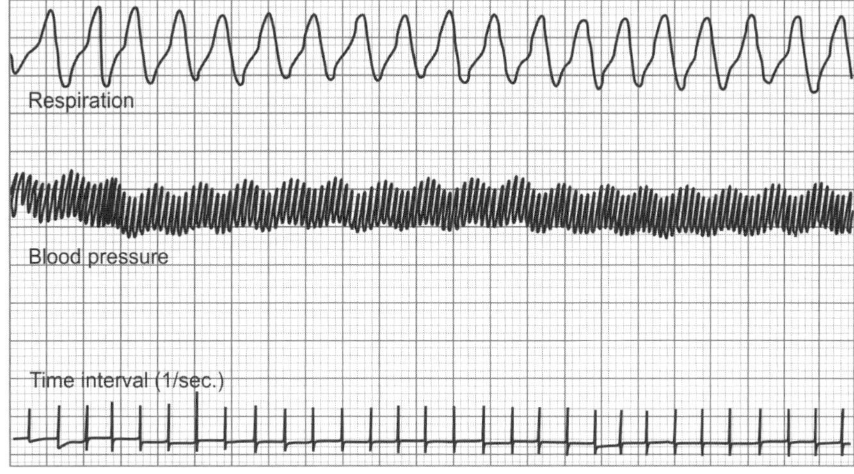

Fig. 6.1: Recording of normal blood pressure and respiration in rabbit

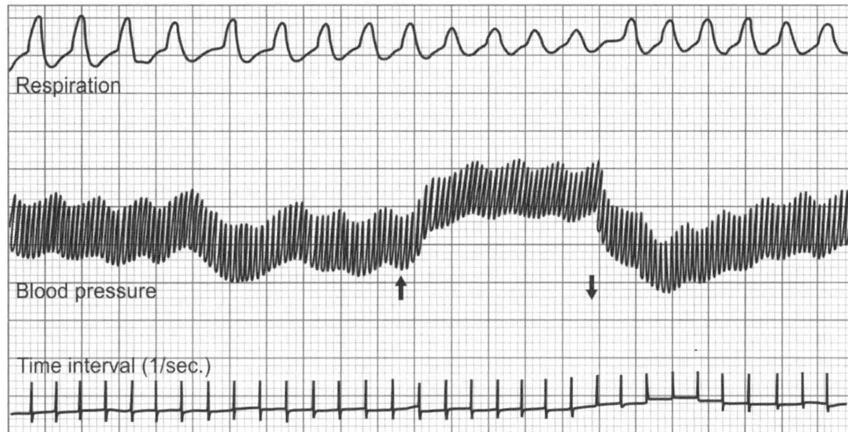

Fig. 6.2: Effect of unilateral occlusion of common carotid artery on blood pressure and respiration in rabbit

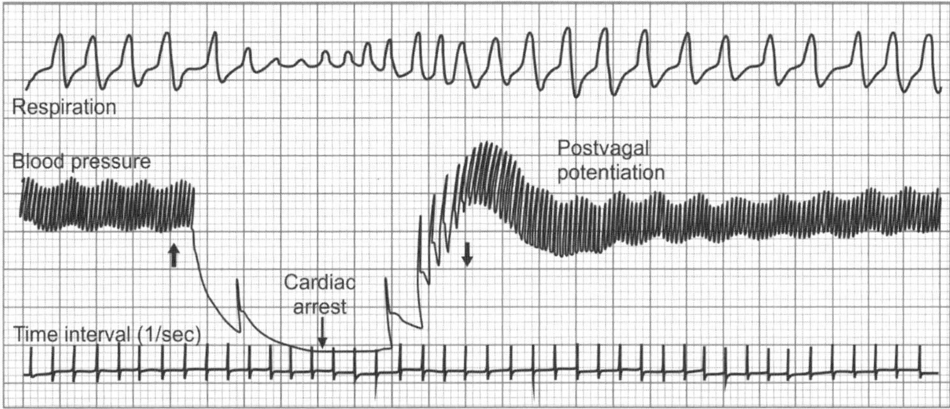

Fig. 6.3: Effect of stimulation of intact vagus nerve on blood pressure and respiration in rabbit. Stimulus parameters: Frequency of stimulation = 30 Hz; Intensity of stimulation = 20 V

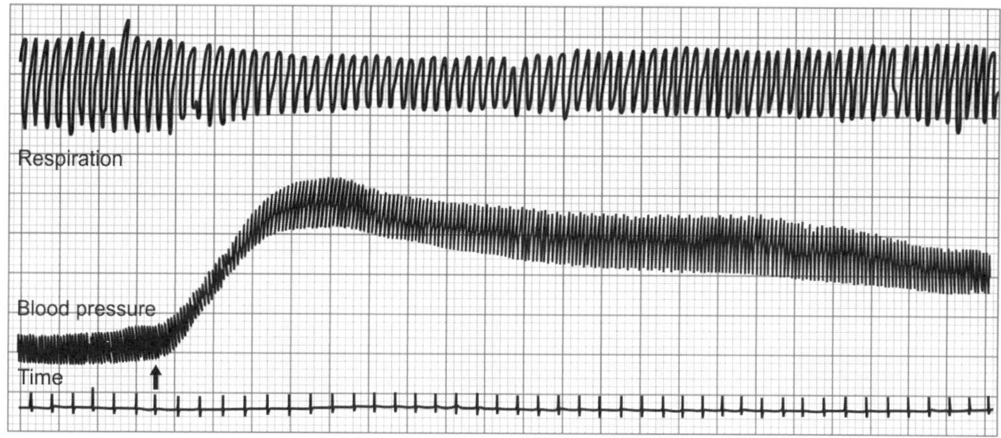

Fig. 6.4: Effect of sympathomimetic drug (adrenaline) on blood pressure and respiration in rabbit.
Dose: 25 µg, IV

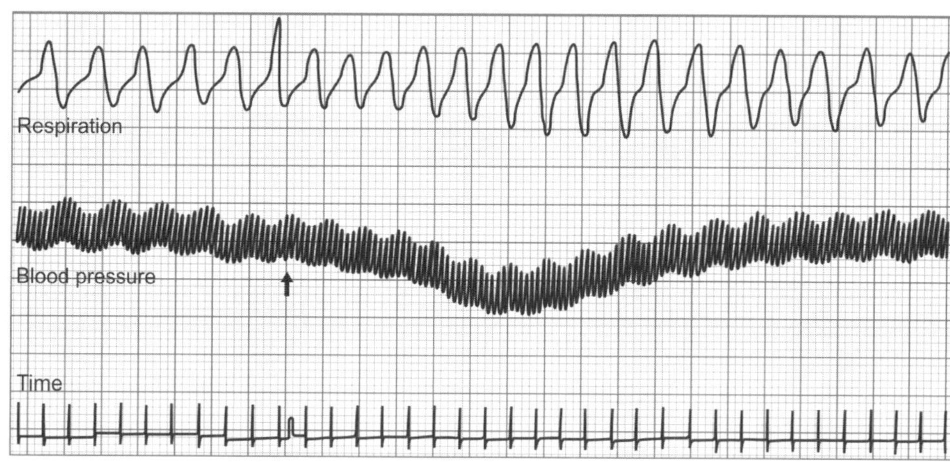

Fig. 6.5: Effect of parasympathomimetic drug (acetylcholine) on blood pressure and respiration in rabbit.
Dose: 10 µg, IV
↑ indicates administration of drug

DEMONSTRATION NO. 2

AIM: TO PERFORM THE PERFUSION OF ISOLATED MAMMALIAN HEART AND TO STUDY THE EFFECT OF DRUGS AND IONS

Equipments

Langendorff's apparatus, Physiograph, Ringer Locke's solution, various Drugs and ions

Langendorff's Apparatus

It consists of a water bath fitted with a heating rod and a thermostat to heat up the water present in the water bath and to keep the temperature constant at 37°C. It also has a stirrer for uniform circulation of warm water. A reservoir bottle (Mariotte bottle) with an attached side tube is present above the water bath. This side tube is connected through a rubber tubing to a coiled glass tube kept in the water bath. This reservoir bottle and glass tube system is meant for the storage and circulation of Ringer Locke's solution. A four way cannula is attached to free end of the coiled glass tube with help of a rubber tubing.

Procedure

- The water bath is filled with water. The heating rod and the thermostat are switched on.
- The reservoir bottle is filled with Ringer Locke's solution and O_2 is continuously bubbled through it.
- A rabbit is stunned, the thorax is opened and the heart is quickly cleared from all its attachments preserving at least 1 cm length of aorta and this isolated heart preparation is taken out.
- The heart is quickly shifted to chilled Ringer Locke's solution kept in petri dish. It is squeezed to remove any blood clots and also cleared off the attached tissue if any.
- The nozzle of the four way cannula is inserted into aorta of the isolated heart preparation and the heart is tied there with a thread taking care that it should not pierce the aortic valve.
- The perfusion of heart with Ringer Locke's solution is started while maintaining a perfusion pressure of 60–80 mmHg.
- The apex of the heart is connected through a hook and thread passing over the pulleys, to the force transducer attached to a Physiograph.
- The normal cardiogram is recorded.

Effect of Drugs and Ions (Figs 6.6 and 6.7)

The effect of following drugs and ions on heart rate and force contraction is recorded by putting the drug into the rubber tube between the coiled glass tube and four way cannula.

1. Adrenaline—1:100,000 (i.e. 1µg/mL)—1 mL is injected
2. Acetylcholine—1:100,000 (i.e. 10 µg/mL)—0.5 mL is injected
3. Atropine sulphate 1:2,000 (i.e. 0.5 mg/mL)—1 mL is injected
4. 1% NaCl—1 mL
5. 1% KCl—1 mL
6. 1% $CaCl_2$—1 mL.

Questions

1. Give the composition of Ringer Locke's solution and significance of its constituents.
2. Explain the effect of various ions on the isolated heart preparation.

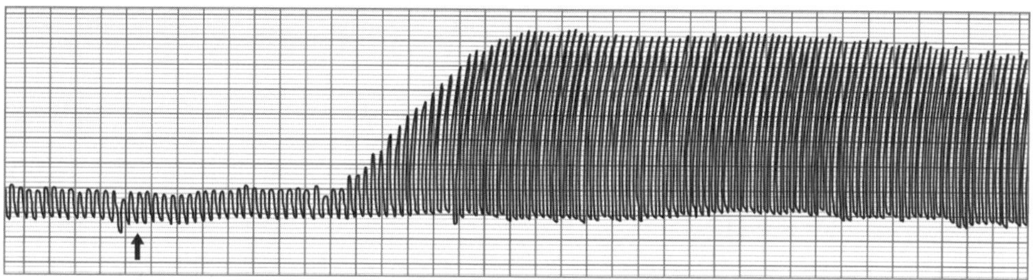

Fig. 6.6: Effect of adrenaline on isolated heart of rabbit. Dose: 1 mL of 1:100,000

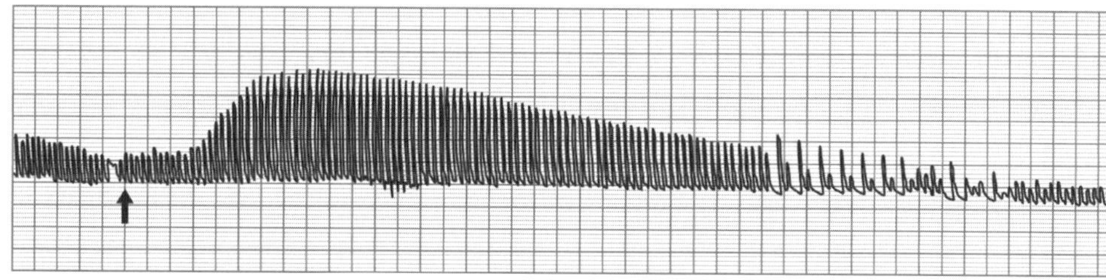

Fig. 6.7: Effect of $CaCl_2$ on isolated heart of rabbit. Dose: 1 mL of 1% $CaCl_2$

DEMONSTRATION NO. 3

AIM: TO RECORD THE MOVEMENTS OF ISOLATED MAMMALIAN INTESTINE AND TO STUDY THE EFFECT OF DRUGS AND IONS

Equipments

Dales Organ Bath, Tyrode solution, Frontal lever, Kymograph

Dales Organ Bath

It consists of:

- A water bath fitted with a heating rod and a thermostat.
- A central glass organ bath of 20 ml capacity with an outlet at its lower end below the water bath.
- A hollow bent glass tube which is curved at the lower end for tying one end of the isolated intestine. This glass tube is fitted in the central glass organ bath. The other end of the tube is used to circulate O_2 into the central glass organ bath.

Procedure

- Water is filled in water bath, heated to 37°C and kept at this temperature with help of the thermostat.
- The organ bath is filled with Tyrode solution and oxygen is continuously bubbled through the Tyrode solution.
- A rabbit is stunned, its abdomen is opened and a part of jejunum close to the duodenum is removed after being cleared of its mesentry and transferred in the Tyrode solution kept in petri dishes.
- The part of intestine removed is cut into 5–6 small segments of 2–3 cm each.
- Lumen of the intestine is cleared by pushing Tyrode solution through the lumen with the help of a syringe.
- A thread is passed through one end of the wall of intestinal segment with help of a stitching needle. A loop of this thread is made to attach the intestine to curved end of the bent glass tube.
- The thread is passed through the wall of the other end of the intestinal segment also in a similar way except that a long thread is kept free for attachment to the frontal lever.
- After some time, intestinal movements can be observed and recorded on drum of the Kymograph moving at a speed of 2.5 mm/second.
- After recording the normal movements the effect of following drugs and ions is observed on the rate and the force of contraction of the intestinal muscle.
  a. Acetylcholine (1:100,000), i.e. 10 µg/ml–1 ml is put in the central glass organ bath
  b. Adrenaline (1:100,000), i.e. 10 µg/ml–0.5 ml is given
  c. 1% $CaCl_2$—1 ml is given
  d. 1% $BaCl_2$—Only a few drops are given
  e. Acetylcholine after atropinization with 1 ml of 0.01% (i.e. 100 µg/ml) of atropine
- After observing the effect of one drug/ion, it should be washed off by repeatedly replacing the Tyrode solution inside the inner organ bath before observing the effect of another drug or ion.

Precautions

1. Freshly prepared and well oxygenated Tyrode solution should always be used.
2. Temperature maintenance at 37° is must for proper working of the preparation.
3. Minimal manual handling of intestinal segment should be done as it may affect motility.

Questions

1. Give the composition of Tyrode solution and significance of its constituents.
2. What types of movements are recorded with this preparation? Comment on various types of intestinal movements.

Chapter

7

Haematology Experiments

AUTHORS

K Sri Nageswari MD FABMS IFME
Professor, Department of Physiology
Dr VRK Women's Medical College
Hyderabad, Telangana, India

Formerly Professor and Head
Department of Physiology
Professor In-Charge–Academics
Government Medical College
Chandigarh, India

Anamika Kothari
Medical Officer
Central Scientific Instruments Organisation (CSIO)
Chandigarh, India

EXPERIMENT NO. 1

AIM: 1. TO UNDERSTAND THE WORKING PRINCIPLE OF MICROSCOPES IN GENERAL

2. TO STUDY COMPOUND MICROSCOPE IN DETAIL

Working of Microscope

Magnification

It is defined as the power of enlargement of an object that cannot be viewed by the naked eye and is done by the microscope so as to see clearly and distinctly the details and contours of closely placed structures of an object.

$$M = \frac{\text{Size of an object/image observed under microscope}}{\text{Actual size of an object}}$$

Resolution

It is defined as the ability to distinguish two closely located points as distinct.

Resolution Power

It is the minimum distance at which two close points can be seen as separate so as to improve the details of an image. It is also known as limit of resolution. Resolution power of unaided human eye is 1/60 of a degree/or 100 mm.

$$Lm = \frac{0.61 \times \lambda}{NA}$$ where, Lm is limit of resolution, λ is wavelength of light.

Resolution power of a lens depends upon wavelength of light and numerical aperture of lens. It can be increased by increasing numerical aperture and decreasing the wavelength of light. NA is numerical aperture of lens.

$NA = n \text{ sine } \alpha$

where, n is refractive index of the medium and sine α is sine of semi-angle of light passing through the objective lens from the specimen. Numerical aperture can be increased by increasing the refractive index of the medium. Refractive index of air, oil immersion lens and most of the optical articles is 1.0,1.5 and 1.6 respectively. Oil immersion objective has more numerical aperture and hence resolution power. Numerical aperture of objective is fixed and that of condenser can be varied by increasing or decreasing the amount of light through the material under observation. It can be done by:

a. By moving the condenser to the uppermost or lowermost position.
b. By operating the iris diaphragm (opening or closing).

Working Distance

- It is the distance between the front surface of the objective lens and the surface of cover glass or the object to be seen. Magnification increases with decrease in working distance.
- Working distance for oil immersion objective is 0.15–1.5 mm

- High power objective is 0.5–4 mm
- Low power objective is 5–15 mm.

Types of Microscopes

There are four types of microscopes depending upon the sources of illumination

a. Light microscope
b. Electron microscope
c. Ultraviolet microscope
d. X-ray microscope

There are various types of Light Microscopes e.g. *Compound, Phase Contrast, Dark Field and Differential Interference Microscope.*

Light (Optical) Microscope (Bright Field Microscope)

Principle: It uses light as a source of illumination and lens for magnification of images so as to reveal details of their structures.

In Compound Microscope, glass lenses are used in combination for magnification.

Phase Contrast Microscope

Discovered by Zernike in 1932.

Principle: Various components of cells refract the light to different degrees. This Microscope multiplies the small differences among the phases or refractive indices of different constituents as well as between the cell interior and outside. It converts these differences of refractive indices into differences of brightness of light.

Refractive index is the degree of light velocity retarded by a substance due to its thickness and opacity.

Uses: It is used to study cells and their constituents in the living state and various physical changes during cellular events e.g. spindle formation, *karyokinesis, cytokinesis, pinocytosis phagocytosis, spermatogenesis* etc.

Dark Field Microscope

Discovered by Zsigmondy in 1903.

Principle: The object is illuminated by oblique beam of light which becomes brightly visible against a dark background e.g. cell organelles, bacteria.

Uses: It is used to see the living objects of less than 0.3 mm. It has a special condenser. There is a disc called stop in the centre of the condenser. As the disc/stop does not allow the light to pass, the central field remains dark.

Differential Interference Microscope

Discovered by Nomarski, 1952.

Principle: The image of the living structures appears as stained due to colour contrast produced by the prism.

In this microscope, two beams of light arising from same source are separated by means of two prisms.

The beam that passes through the object undergoes diffraction or phase change. The second beam travels besides the object which does not undergo any change. These two beams come together above the object and give bright contrast.

Uses: Differential interference microscope gives information about
1. Thickness of the objects.
2. Presence of various light absorbing materials like nucleic acids, proteins, lipids etc. and gives better images as compared to phase contrast microscope.

Fluorescent Microscope

Discovered by Coons in 1941.

Principle: A tissue stained with fluorescent dye absorbs radiation of short wavelength i.e. ultraviolet radiation, gets excited and emits back light energy of long wavelength, which is in the visible spectrum and is seen by fluorescent microscope.

Uses: It is used in immunological laboratories .The substances, which can emit fluorescence, when excited by short wavelength light can be used for tagging cellular components and are known as Fluorochromes e.g. acridine orange, FITC.

Electron Microscope

Principle: In Electron Microscope, three electromagnets are used in place of glass lenses i.e. condenser, objective and projector. A beam of electrons is made to pass through high vacuum for illumination of object and image formation. There are two types of electron microscopes
1. Transmission electron microscope: It was invented by Knoll and Ruska in 1931. It magnifies the image 100,000 -300,000 times and resolution power is 1-10A°.
2. Scanning electron microscope: It was discovered by Knoll in 1935. It has magnification range up to 200,000. Resolution 10 nm.

Uses: It is employed in the study of ultra structure of cells and small structures like spores and microorganisms.

Compound Microscope in Detail

Compound Microscope was invented by Antonie van Leeuwenhoek in 1674. It is an optical instrument by which objects that are not visible to the naked eye are magnified. It consists of:
1. *The stand or base:* It comprises of a heavy foot and is connected to the handle, which bears the optical system. It gives mechanical stability to the instrument. It supports the microscope on working table.
2. *Handle:* It is curved and the microscope can be tilted at the hinge when desired.
3. *Tube:* It is a cylindrical tube through which light traverses. Its length determines the mechanical length of the microscope (mechanical length is the distance between upper part of the objective and eye piece). It consists of two parts:
   a. *Outer or external tube:* It bears nosepiece at lower end of the tube to which three objective lenses are fitted
      - Low power 10×
      - High power 40×
      - Oil immersion 100×

   b. *Inner tube:* It carries the eyepiece at its upper end having magnification of 5× or 10×. Inner tube can slide inside the outer tube to adjust the mechanical length. Normally it is 160 mm.
4. *Fine and coarse adjustment*: With help of these adjustments, height of the tube can be adjusted so that the objective lens can be positioned at its optimal distance (focal length) so that the object can be examined. A third knob is there to move condenser.
5. *The stage*: It is a platform on which glass slide is accommodated on which the object is mounted. There is an aperture in the centre to permit light to reach the object.
6. *The sub-stage*: It consists of a condenser and a diaphragm.
   a. *Condenser:* It is a system of lenses, which focuses light from light source on the object. The intensity of illumination of the object can be varied by raising or lowering the condenser. Position of condenser is highest when oil immersion is used and lowest when low power objective lens is used.
   b. *Iris diaphragm:* It controls the amount of light reaching the condenser.
7. *Mirror*: At the foot end of the microscope below the condenser, the hinged double reflecting mirror is fitted, which is plane on one side and concave on the other side. Plane mirror is used when condenser is at the highest position and source of light is diffuse e.g. sunlight. Concave mirror is used when source of light is artificial or limited e.g. bulb or tube light as in laboratory.

Calculation of Magnification of Object

Power of eyepiece × power of objective lens × tube factor

Method of Focusing of an Object

- *Under low power (10 × objective):* Place the slide on the mechanical stage and bring the object near the central aperture in the stage and bring the low power objective above the aperture of stage. Using distant light/artificial light and plane/concave mirror focus the light on the object with condenser in its lowest position. Using coarse adjustment, lower the tube and focus the object. Now with the help of fine adjustment the slide can be brought to a sharp focus.
- *Under high power (40 × objective):* Revolve the nosepiece clockwise to bring the high power objective near the central aperture of the stage. Condenser is raised. Iris diaphragm is fully opened and concave mirror is used to focus artificial light on the object under observation. The object is finally focused using fine adjustment.
- *Oil immersion (100 × objective):* Revolve the nosepiece to bring oil immersion objective above the object. Raise the tube and a drop of cedar wood oil is placed on the area of the slide to be focused. Lower the tube again till the objective just touches the drop of oil. Iris diaphragm is fully opened and condenser is in top position. Then using fine adjustment, focus the area to be examined.

Precautions

- Eye piece as well as objectives should be cleaned after every use
- Always clean the objectives with xylene, not with alcohol as alcohol may dissolve the cement used in component of lenses
- Never lower the tube quickly while looking through the eyepiece

- As the tube is lowered using coarse adjustment, visualise from the side so that the coarse adjustment is stopped as the objective just touches the drop of oil. This step is taken to prevent the damage to the objective especially with high power and oil immersion lens
- Care should be taken while handling the microscope. (Always hold upright by handling with a hand below its base).

QUESTIONS

1. Describe the principle of microscopy and explain resolution.
2. Explain the numerical aperture and working distance in microscopy and its relation to magnification.
3. What are different adjustments made in the microscope while using different types of objectives and sources of light?
4. Enumerate the functions of condenser and iris diaphragm.

EXPERIMENT NO. 2

AIM: COLLECTION OF BLOOD SAMPLE

Principle

When the quantity of blood required is small for investigations such as haemoglobin estimation, TLC, RBC count, DLC, clotting time, blood groups etc. capillary blood is obtained from finger-prick method. For larger quantities of blood as is required for biochemical and hematological tests like PCV, ESR, Osmotic fragility etc., venous blood is obtained from antecubital vein by venipuncture.

Collection of Capillary Blood

Apparatus

1. Disposable sterile lancet/disposable needle
2. Spirit
3. Cotton swab
4. Glass slides or designated pipettes.

Procedure

- Warm the finger to be pricked by rubbing to improve the circulation
- Clean the finger tip with spirit (any of the three middle fingers is used, preferably the ring finger)
- Allow the finger to dry (as spirit will haemolyse the blood)
- Prick the finger sharply and quickly, deep enough so as to allow free flow of blood and the drop appears automatically
- Discard or wipe away one or two drops of the blood as it might contain tissue fluid which dilutes the blood and decreases the estimated values.

Precautions

- Use disposable lancet and do not touch its tip
- Do not use same needle for different individuals. If the same needle is being used then sterilise and clean it with spirit before reuse
- Allow the finger to dry after cleaning with spirit
- Do not squeeze the finger as tissue fluid will dilute the blood
- Discard first one or two drops
- Middle three fingers are to be used because bursae of thumb and little finger are continuous with that of the forearm whereas bursae of middle three fingers are limited to the hand only.

Collection of Venous Sample

Apparatus

1. Disposable syringe and needle
2. Spirit

3. Cotton swab
4. Collection vial or glass tube with anticoagulant.

Procedure

- Procedure is explained to the subject and his/her consent is taken
- After location of a vein in antecubital fossa (as median cubital vein is commonly used for puncture), arm is to be supported on the edge of the table
- Tourniquet is to be applied just above the elbow and the subject is asked to clench his/her fist
- Skin over the vein is cleaned with spirit swab after feeling for the vein by the index finger
- Skin over the vein is stretched downwards and needle is inserted and pushed gently along the line of vein for a small distance and blood is withdrawn
- Tourniquet is removed, while the needle is still in the vein
- Needle is gently removed after placing the spirit swab on the obscured part of the needle
- Needle is removed from the syringe and blood is poured into the vial or tube having anticoagulant
- After collection of the sample, the spirit swab should be kept pressed against the punctured site for few minutes so as to avoid oozing/bleeding.

Precautions

- Collection vial containing anticoagulant should be kept ready before starting the procedure
- The consent should be obtained and the subject should be seated comfortably
- Aseptic precautions should be taken at all stages
- Disposable syringes and needles should be used
- Vein should be made prominent and visible before making puncture
- Tourniquet should be removed before taking needle out of the vein to prevent haematoma formation
- To prevent clotting blood should be immediately transferred to vial/tube containing the anticoagulant.

Anticoagulants

Anticoagulants prevent clotting:

- *EDTA (Ethylenediaminetetraacetic acid)*: The sodium and potassium salts of EDTA are powerful anticoagulants. Di-potassium salts are preferred as they are more soluble. It acts by chelating calcium in the blood. Anhydrous salt (1.2 mg) of EDTA is used per ml of blood. Excess of EDTA causes shrinkage and destruction of cells, significant decrease in PCV by centrifugation and increases MCHC. Platelets are also disintegrated and give increased platelet count.

  Uses: Routine hematological procedures except coagulation studies.
- *Sodium Citrate:* It acts by chelating calcium ions. One volume of sodium citrate is added to 9 volumes of blood for coagulation studies. It is used for estimation of ESR in 4:1 ratio (4 volumes of blood is added to 1 volume of sodium citrate) by Westergren method.
- *Double Oxalate:* It forms insoluble complex with calcium in blood and inhibit coagulation. It is used for estimation of ESR, PCV and investigations in which volume of the cells should not be affected.

- *Heparin:* It acts by inhibiting thrombin and other stages of clotting factor activation. It is used at a concentration of 10-20 IU/ml of blood. It is also used for blood gas determination and pH assays and is best for osmotic fragility. It should not be used for leucocyte count as it causes clumping of leucocytes and gives blue colour to the background in DLC.
- *ACD:* Acid citrate dextrose used in blood bank as an anticoagulant.

QUESTIONS

1. Enumerate various anticoagulants and give a note on their mode of action.
2. Differentiate between peripheral and venous blood.

EXPERIMENT NO. 3

AIM: PREPARATION AND STAINING OF PERIPHERAL BLOOD SMEAR

Apparatus and Reagents

1. Compound microscope
2. Glass slides
3. Spreader
4. Sterile pricking needle (disposable)
5. Leishman's stain
6. Buffer
7. Cedar wood oil
8. Cotton and spirit.

Leishman's Stain

It is Romanowsky group of stain consisting of:

a. 10% solution of methylene blue prepared in 0.5% Na_2CO_3
b. Equal volume of 0.1% solution of eosin is added
c. The solution is dried and powdered
d. 0.15 gm of the powder is dissolved in 100 ml of acetone free methyl alcohol.

Eosin: It is an acidic dye and stains granules of eosinophils and haemoglobin of RBC.

Methylene blue: It is a basic dye, stains RNA of cytoplasm, DNA of nuclei and granules of basophils.

Acetone free methyl alcohol: It fixes the smear to the glass slide.

Buffer Solution

Buffer is the fluid that consists of a weak acid and its salt or a weak base and its salt that has the ability to maintain pH of the solution.

Iso-osmotic Phosphate Buffer

It consists of:

- Solution A: NaH_2PO_4—23.4 g/l
- Solution B: Na_2HPO_4—21.3 g/l

Phosphate Buffer solution of desired pH can be prepared by adding different quantities of Na_2HPO_4 and NaH_2PO_4 solutions.

pH	*Solution A*	*Solution B*
5.8	87 ml	13 ml
6.0	83 ml	17 ml
6.2	75 ml	25 ml
6.4	66 ml	34 ml
6.6	56 ml	44 ml

pH	*Solution A*	*Solution B*
6.8	46 ml	54 ml
7.0	32 ml	68 ml
7.2	24 ml	76 ml
7.4	18 ml	82 ml
7.6	13 ml	87 ml
7.7	9.5 ml	90.5 ml

Preparation of Blood Smear (Wedge Method)

- Clean and grease free glass slides (3-4) and a spreader with smooth edges are taken
- The slide as well as the spreading edge are marked
- The tip of ring or middle finger of left hand is cleaned with spirit and allowed to dry
- The finger is pricked with sterile lancet and a drop of blood is allowed to form
- The first drop is discarded (as it might contain tissue fluid) and a reasonable sized drop of blood is obtained
- Blood drop is placed on one end of the glass slide about 1 cm away from the edge
- The slide is placed on flat surface of the table and the smooth edge of spreader is held just in front of the drop at an angle of 45°
- The spreader is drawn backwards so that it just touches the drop and the blood is allowed to spread along the edge of the spreader
- Spreader is then moved towards the other end of the slide smoothly and slowly (maintaining the even pressure and at 45° angle) so as to prepare a smear
- Immediately the smear is dried in the air
- The procedure is repeated till ideal film is obtained.

Criteria of Good Blood Smear

- Smear should occupy 3–4 cm length of the slide/middle 2/3rd of slide
- It should be tongue shaped with no tails at the end (It has three parts head, body and tail)
- Thickness should be uniform. It should not be too thick or too thin, no longitudinal or cross striations should be visible under microscope
- There should be no interruptions in between
- There should be no collection of blood at either ends
- It should be one cell thick when visualised under microscope and cells should be uniformly distributed.

Staining of Blood Smear

- The slide is placed on stand/rod in horizontal position
- Leishman's stain (8–12 drops) is poured on slide so that it just covers the smear fully
- It is kept for two minutes. This is to fix the smear on the slide. This is known as fixation time
- Equal drops of buffer (pH 7.4) are added and mixed thoroughly by blowing air from side gently
- Waiting time of 5–10 minutes is given. During this time the smear is actually stained. This is known as staining time

- Proper staining procedure gives a green scum over the stain
- The slide is washed with tap water (taking care that water stream should not strike smear directly)
- The slide is kept vertically for drying
- Properly stained slide should look bluish pink
- The smear is dried and examined under low and high power and then under oil immersion of the microscope.

Criteria of Well-stained Smear

- A well-stained smear looks bluish pink on naked eye examination
- Under low and high power objectives of the microscope, we can examine for quality of the smear
- RBCs: Look orange pink/buff colour, one cell layer thick and uniformly distributed
- WBCs: At least one WBC per high power field
- Overstaining: RBCs look blue
WBCs look bluish black (dark)
- Understaining: RBCs are pale
WBCs are colourless

Precautions

- Slide should be clean and grease free
- The surface of the glass slide should be marked with glass marking pencil
- The spreading edge of the spreader should be smooth as it will otherwise cause tail in the smear and gives rise to uneven distribution of the cells
- The spreader is used for six times only
- The smear is dried immediately (do not dry with heat)
- Maintaining an angle of 45° between slide and spreader (if the angle is more than 45° thick smear will result and lesser angle gives thin smear), the smear is drawn
- Smear should be stained within two hours
- Sufficient time is allowed for fixation of smear. Staining time depends upon strength of Leishman's stain and varies with each batch of stain
- After staining, smear is washed properly and water stream should not strike smear directly
- If slide is under stained, repeat the process for few minutes and if it is over stained wash it again for few minutes.

QUESTIONS

1. Mention the clinical significance of peripheral blood smear.
2. Describe the composition of Buffer and its function.
3. What is the composition of Leishman's stain and mention the functions subserved by each of its constituents.

EXPERIMENT NO. 4

AIM: DIFFERENTIAL LEUCOCYTE COUNT

Differential Leucocyte Count (DLC)

It denotes the percentage of different types of white blood cells in the blood.

Apparatus and Reagents

1. Microscope
2. Glass slides
3. Spreader
4. Cotton
5. Spirit
6. Sterile finger pricking needle
7. Leishman's stain
8. Cedar wood oil
9. Buffer (7.4).

Procedure

- The finger is pricked using aseptic precautions
- A well-stained smear is prepared and examined for quality of smear under low and high power of microscope
- Identification and counting of different types of leucocytes is done under oil immersion keeping the following morphological features in mind:
  a. Size.
  b. Nucleus: Staining reaction, number of lobes, chromatin structure
  c. Cytoplasm: Colour, granules and characteristics
  d. Nucleus to cytoplasmic ratio.
- A minimum of 100 leucocytes are counted using tally bar method to avoid recounting of the same cell.

Tally Bar Method

The cells are counted from the head end of the smear along a longitudinal strip towards the tail and then by moving two fields down, the film is scanned in the opposite direction, again moving two fields down as the other end is approached. Examine the smear in this fashion till 100 cells are counted.

Percentage of Different Leucocytes*

Neutrophils	–	40–75%
Eosinophils	–	1–6%
Basophils	–	0–1%
Lymphocytes	–	20–50%
Monocytes	–	2–10%

* Values from reference No. 3

Causes of Neutrophilia

Physiological Causes

- *After food intake*
- *Exercise*
- *Stress*
- *Pregnancy and parturition*
- *Exposure to cold.*

Pathological Causes

- *Acute pyogenic infections*
- *Tissue injuries e.g. trauma, surgery, burns, infarction*
- *Haemorrhage*
- *Inflammatory conditions e.g. rheumatic fever, collagen disorders*
- *Leukaemia*
- *Metabolic disorders e.g. diabetic ketoacidosis, hepatic coma, uraemia*
- *Steroid therapy.*

Types of leucocytes (Figs 7, Plate 4)**

	Size	*Nucleus*	*Cytoplasm*
A. Granulocytes			
1. Neutrophils	10–15 μm	2–5 lobed, connected by chromatin filaments, purplish blue	Colour of the cytoplasm is light purple/ faint pink. Granules are fine and stain purple
2. Eosinophils	10–15 μm	Bilobed or trilobed connected with chromatin strands (spectacle appearance), Purplish blue	Cytoplasm is pink in colour. Brick red coarse granules (pearl drop appearance)
3. Basophils	10–15 μm	Bilobed or S shaped, Purplish blue	Cytoplasm is blue. Scanty and coarse granules, deep ink blue, completely masking the nucleus
B. Agranulocytes			
1. Monocytes	15–20 μm	Single large, deeply convoluted nucleus, eccentric, pale bluish violet	Abundant cytoplasm. Ground glass appearance. Sometimes azurophilic granules are seen. Colour of cytoplasm is grayish/cloudy blue
2. Small lymphocyte	6–8 μm	Single large nucleus almost completely filling the cell, compact deep purplish blue (ink dot appearance)	Scanty, light violet/sky blue in colour
3. Large lymphocyte	10–15 μm	Single large centrally placed, kidney shaped nucleus filling the cell and staining deep purplish blue	Less amount of cytoplasm, light violet/sky blue colour
***Compiled from various practical physiology and clinical haematology books as per given references*			

Causes of Neutropenia

Physiological

- *Infants (40% is the normal count)*
- *Exposure to severe cold.*

Pathological

1. *Due to increased utilisation*
   - Infections e.g. typhoid, early stages of viral infections
   - Over-whelming sepsis (where consumption of neutrophils exceeds production).
2. *Due to ineffective leucopoiesis*
   - Aplastic anaemia (due to suppression of myeloid cells)
   - Drug-induced neutropenia (due to suppression of granulocytic precursors e.g. anti-cancerous drugs, phenothiazines, sulpha drugs, phenylbutazone)
   - Deficiency of vitamin B_{12} and folic acid results in defective synthesis of DNA
   - Starvation
   - Leukaemia and lymphoma (due to replacement of normal hemopoietic tissue in bone marrow by neoplastic cells).
3. *Accelerated removal or destruction*
   - Immunological injury e.g. Felty's syndrome
   - Hypersplenism
   - Megaloblastic anaemia (deficiency of vitamin B_{12} and folic acid results in defective DNA synthesis which produces abnormal precursors rendering them susceptible to death).

Lymphocytosis

Physiological

Infants (40–60% is the normal count).

Pathological

- *Chronic infections e.g. Tuberculosis, Syphilis, Brucellosis*
- *Viral infections e.g. hepatitis, Whooping cough, Infectious mononucleosis, Cytomegalovirus infection*
- *Lymphocytic leukaemia.*

Lymphopenia

- *Infections e.g. Acquired immune deficiency syndrome*
- *ACTH therapy and immunosuppressive therapy*
- *Hodgkin's disease*
- *Bone marrow suppression*

Monocytosis

- *Protozoal diseases e.g. Malaria, Kala-azar*

- *Viral diseases e.g. Infectious mononucleosis*
- *Chronic infections e.g. Tuberculosis, Syphilis, Rickettsia etc.*
- *Acute bacterial endocarditis*
- *Monocytic leukaemia*
- *ACTH therapy*
- *Granulocytic disorders, e.g. Sarcoidosis, Ulcerative colitis, Regional enteritis*
- *Collagen disorders e.g. Systemic lupus erythematosus, Rheumatoid arthritis.*

Monocytopenia

- *Bone marrow suppression*
- *Septicaemia.*

Eosinophilia

- *Allergic conditions e.g. Food and drug allergy, Bronchial asthma, Hay fever, Urticaria*
- *Parasitic infestations e.g. Ascariasis, Hookworm disease, Hydatid disease, Filariasis*
- *Dermatological conditions e.g. Pemphigus, Psoriasis*
- *Dermatitis herpetiformis*
- *Leukaemias*
- *Collagen disorders*
- *Post-splenectomy*
- *Hodgkin's disease.*

Eosinopenia

- *Aplastic anaemia*
- *ACTH therapy*
- *Cushing's disease.*

Basophilia

- *Chronic myeloid leukaemia*
- *Polycythaemia.*

Basopenia

- *Severe septicaemia*
- *Aplastic anaemia.*

QUESTIONS

1. Mention the clinical significance of differential leucocyte count.
2. How does the DLC of a child differ from that of an adult?
3. Enumerate the functions of leucocytes.

EXPERIMENT NO. 5

AIM: TO PREPARE A PERIPHERAL BLOOD SMEAR AND PERFORM COOKE-ARNETH COUNT

Cooke-Arneth Count

It is the counting of neutrophils (100–200) and expressing the result in terms of number of lobes of their nuclei.

Apparatus and Reagents

1. Microscope
2. Glass slides
3. Cover slip
4. Sterile pricking needle
5. Spirit
6. Cotton
7. Leishman's stain
8. Cedar wood oil and Buffer.

Procedure (Tally Bar Method)

- The finger is pricked using aseptic precautions
- A well-stained blood smear is made
- The smear is examined under low and high power of the microscope for ensuring proper quality of the smear and distribution of cells
- The smear is examined under oil immersion and 100–200 neutrophils are counted noting the number of lobes of the nucleus in each cell
- The percentage of cells in each stage is calculated.

Normal Values*

Stage I (N1)	Single lobed	Nucleus is C shaped	5–10%
Stage II (N2)	Bilobed	2 lobes are connected by chromatin filaments	20–30%
Stage III (N3)	Trilobed	3 lobes are connected by chromatin filaments	40–50%
Stage IV (N4)	Tetralobed	4 lobes connected by chromatin filaments	10–15%
Stage V (N5,6)	Five lobed	5 or more lobes connected by chromatin filaments	3–5%

Clinical Significance

Left shift (Regenerative shift) N1+N2+N3 >80%
Indicates hyperactive bone marrow.

* Values from reference no. 1

Right shift (Degenerative shift) N4+N5+N6 >20%
Indicates hypoactive bone marrow.

Causes of Shift to Left

- *Acute pyogenic infections*
- *Tuberculosis (due to increased destruction of older neutrophils)*
- *Haemorrhage*
- *Radiation (low doses)*
- *Leukaemias.*

Causes of Shift to Right

- *Megaloblastic anaemia*
- *Aplastic anaemia*
- *Septicaemia*
- *Uraemia*
- *High doses of radiation*
- *Agranulocytosis due to drugs*
  - Chloramphenicol
  - Anticancer drugs e.g. cyclophosphamide
  - Methotrexate.

QUESTION

1. Mention the significance of Cooke-Arneth count and explain the relationship of nuclear lobes with the age of neutrophils.

EXPERIMENT NO. 6

AIM: ESTIMATION OF HAEMOGLOBIN USING SAHLI'S METHOD

Principle

The haemoglobin in the blood is converted into acid hematin by the action of N/10 HCl, which is brown in colour. The intensity of colour of the solution depends upon the amount of acid haematin, which in turn depends on the haemoglobin concentration. The colour is matched against standard brown tinted glass filters/rods, which gives the reading in gm/100 ml of blood and also in percentage.

Apparatus and Reagents

1. *Sahli's haemoglobinometer consists of:*
   a. *Haemoglobin tube:* It is a square or round tube graduated in 2-22 g% and percentage (10–140%).
   b. *Haemoglobin pipette:* It is a straight glass capillary pipette with single mark i.e. 20 cumm. There is no bulb as no dilution of blood is required.
   c. *A glass rod stirrer:* It is provided for mixing blood with acid solution. The broader end, which is like spatula, should be used for stirring.
   d. *Comparator box:* It is a rectangular box with a slot in centre, which accommodates the haemoglobin tube. On either side of the slot are two solid standard brown glass rods/filter. A white opaque glass is fitted behind the slot to provide necessary background and permit uniform illumination during colour matching.
2. *N/10 HCl:* It is prepared by adding 3.65 gm HCl in 1 liter of distilled water.
3. Distilled water for dilution.
4. Dropper.
5. Sterile pricking apparatus, cotton and spirit.

Procedure

- With the help of dropper, graduated haemoglobin tube is filled with N/10 HCl up to the mark 20% or 3 gm%
- The finger is pricked using aseptic precautions and first drop is wiped off and a drop of blood of reasonable size is obtained
- The haemoglobin pipette is held close to the tip of the drop and blood is drawn up to 20 mm^3 mark into the pipette (taking care that no air bubble should be drawn) and the extra blood adhering to the tip and sides, if any, is wiped off
- Immediately the blood is transferred into the haemoglobin tube and mixed well with stirrer
- The solution is left for 10 minutes for conversion of haemoglobin to acid haematin
- Distilled water is added drop by drop, mixing it thoroughly each time with the stirrer and matching the colour against standard glass each time
- The reading is noted by taking lower meniscus of the solution in gm%. The stirrer should be lifted just above the solution but not completely out of the tube while matching and taking the reading. The matching should be carried out against enough light/day light

- Since the colour may seem to match over a wide range of dilutions, so as to avoid the error (which is 10–15%), it is advisable to take three readings:
  - Ist reading: When the colour of the solution is just one shade dark than the standard glass
  - IInd reading: When it exactly matches the standard glass
  - IIIrd reading: When the colour is one shade lighter than the standard glass

  The average of these three readings is taken.

Normal Values

Male	–	13.5–18 g%
Female	–	11.5–16 g%
Newborns and Infants	–	18–20 g%

Other Methods

Cyanmethaemoglobin method: Haemoglobin is converted into cyanmethaemoglobin by Drabkin's reagent (sodium bicarbonate 1 gm, potassium cyanide 50 mg, potassium ferricyanide 200 mg and distilled water). Absorbance of the solution is measured in photo colourimeter provided with yellow green filter (540 nm).

Haldane's method: RBC's are haemolysed in hypotonic solution (distilled water) and carbon monoxide is added to the solution and light pink colour of the solution is compared with standard.

Wu method: All forms of haemoglobin are converted into alkaline hematin with NaOH.

Tallquist method: It is quick but inaccurate. Touch the drop of blood with a piece of a filter paper and allow the blood to diffuse to stain the paper. As soon as the colour of the blood stain loses its gloss and before drying, match the colour against printed red coloured spots on a chart representing the various concentrations of haemoglobin in percentage.

Photoelectric colourimetric method (Spectrophotometery): The photoelectric colourimeter measures the amount of light (of limited wave band) absorbed by the solution. The wave band is chosen to correspond to that part of the spectrum that is maximally absorbed by the solution being tested.

$CuSO_4$ falling drop method: A drop of blood is dropped into a solution of Copper Sulphate, which has given specific gravity. The density of drop is directly proportional to the amount of haemoglobin in that drop. If the drop is denser than specific gravity of the solution, the drop sinks and if not, it will float on the top.

Clinical Significance of Haemoglobin

Causes of Increased Haemoglobin Concentration

A. *Errors of procedure*
   - Amount of blood taken in haemoglobin pipette is above mark 20 cmm
   - Faded colour of comparator box.

B. *Due to increased RBC count*

   Physiological causes
   - *Newborn and infants*

- *High altitude*
- *Exercise*
- *Excessive sweating.*

Pathological causes

- *Polycythemia*
- *Chronic hypoxic conditions e.g. congenital heart diseases, lung diseases like Emphysema.*
- *Conditions resulting in haemoconcentration e.g. severe vomiting and diarrhoea.*

Causes of Decreased Haemoglobin Concentration

A. *Errors of procedure*
- Dilution of blood by tissue fluid
- Amount of blood taken below mark 20 mm^3
- Improper mixing of blood resulting in inadequate acid haematin formation
- Inadequate time given for reaction of blood and N/10 HCl.

B. *Due to decreased RBC count*

Physiological causes
- *Infants of 0–3 months of age (due to milk diet)*
- *Females (due to inhibitory effect of oestrogen on erythropoiesis*
- *Pregnancy (due to haemodilution)*
- *Menstruation (loss of blood).*

Pathological causes
- *Anaemias*
- *Haemodilution e.g. ADH secreting pituitary tumour.*

QUESTIONS

1. Describe the various methods for estimating haemoglobin.
2. Why any strong acid or alkali cannot be used to hemolyse the RBC for estimation of haemoglobin?
3. Enumerate the different reactions of haemoglobin.

EXPERIMENT NO. 7

AIM: TOTAL LEUCOCYTE COUNT

Principle

A known volume of blood is diluted with Turk's fluid (1 in 20 dilution) which haemolyses the red blood cells and stains the nuclei of WBC. Total numbers of leucocytes are calculated per mm^3 of undiluted blood using dilution factor.

Composition of Turk's Fluid

a. Glacial acetic acid 1% (It haemolyses RBCs)
b. Gentian violet 0.3% W/V (stains the nuclei of WBC)
c. Distilled water.

Apparatus

- Microscope
- *Neubauer counting chamber*: It is a thick glass slide divided into two central platforms by an H-shaped groove. Central platform is slightly lower than the sides so that when a cover slip is placed there is a space of 1/10 mm between the cover slip and central platform. Counting area on either side is of 3 mm × 3 mm which is further divided into 9 squares, each measuring 1 mm × 1 mm. Among the nine squares the corner four squares are used for WBC count and central square for RBC count. Each WBC square is further divided into 16 small squares. The area of each WBC square is 1 mm × 1 mm = 1 mm^2. The depth of each WBC square is 1/10 mm. Hence the volume of each square will be 0.1 mm × 1 mm^2 = 0.1 mm^3. Thus the volume of four WBC squares is 0.1 mm^3 × 4 = 0.4mm^3.
- WBC Pipette: It is graduated glass tube with three markings (0.5, 1 and 11) and bulb containing white glass bead
- Cover slip.
- Sterile pricking needle, cotton, spirit.

Procedure

- Pipette, Neubauer chamber and cover slip are cleaned thoroughly
- Finger is pricked under aseptic precautions and first drop is discarded
- Blood is sucked up to mark 0.5 and extra amount of the blood adhering to the tip of the pipette is wiped off
- Turk's fluid is drawn up to mark 11 and mixed thoroughly by rotating the pipette in between the palms keeping the pipette horizontally. A waiting time of 8–10 minutes is given
- Neubauer chamber is placed on the stage of the microscope and WBC squares are brought under focus with low power of the microscope
- Chamber is removed from the microscope stage and a coverslip is placed on the ruled area of the central platform

- First few drops of fluid from pipette are discarded as it contains diluting fluid only
- A drop is allowed to form at the tip of the pipette. Keeping the pipette horizontal, tip of the pipette is touched at the edge of the coverslip at 45° angle
- Diluted blood is allowed to flow under the coverslip by capillary action and pipette is quickly removed
- Cells are allowed to settle down for 2–3 minutes before placing the charged chamber on the stage of the microscope
- The chamber is focused under low power and uniformity of distribution of the cells is checked (if cells are not uniformly distributed, clean the chamber and recharge it)
- WBCs are clear, refractile, nucleated and rounded bodies
- Cells are counted in 4 corner squares (to avoid recounting of the same cells again white blood cells present in the left and upper margins of the square are omitted while cells on right and lower margins are counted or vice versa.

Calculations

1. *Dilution factor:* As 0.5 parts of blood are mixed with 10.5 parts of Turk's fluid, and the initial part of fluid marked '1' remains in the stem of the pipette and does not contain cells, is discarded, this volume is deducted from total volume i.e. 11-1 = 10. Hence 0.5 parts of blood is diluted in 10 parts of fluid and therefore the dilution factor is 1 in 20.
2. WBC count per cubic mm of undiluted blood
   - Area of one WBC square = 1 mm × 1 mm = 1 mm^2
   - Depth of one WBC square = 0.1 mm
   - Volume of 4 WBC squares = 4 × 0.1 mm × 1 mm^2 = 0.4 mm^3
   - Total cells in 0.4 mm^3 volume of diluted blood = N
   - Cells in 1 mm^3 of diluted blood will be = N/0.4

   Therefore, cells in 1 mm^3 of undiluted blood will be = N/0.4 × 20 (dilution factor) = N × 50.

Precautions

- Aseptic procedures are to be followed at all stages
- Pipette, Neubauer chamber and coverslip should be clean and dry
- Blood should be sucked exactly up to mark 0.5 and tip of the pipette is to be wiped off, if any blood is adhering to it
- Diluting fluid should be sucked exactly up to mark 11
- There should be no air bubbles while sucking the fluid/blood in the pipette and while charging the chamber
- Mixing of the blood and fluid should be done thoroughly, keeping the pipette horizontally
- The chamber should not be overcharged (overflow of fluid into the gutters) or undercharged (fluid does not spread on the entire central platform). If the chamber is overcharged, cells may enter into the gutter and settle there and give false results and if it is undercharged cells may not be found in peripheral squares
- After charging, counting should be done as early as possible before fluid begins to dry up
- If distribution of the cells is not uniform chamber should be cleaned and recharged.

Normal Values*

Adults	4,000–11,000/mm^3 of blood
Newborns	10,000–25,000/mm^3 of blood
Infants	6,000–18,000/mm^3 of blood
Children	5,000–15,000/mm^3 of blood

Clinical Significance

Leucocytosis

A. *Physiological*
- Newborns and infants
- Physical exercise
- After food intake
- Increased environmental temperature
- Pregnancy
- Menstruation
- Mental stress
- Parturition.

B. *Pathological*
- Acute bacterial infections
- Tuberculosis
- Tissue injury—burns, surgery, infarction
- Haemorrhage
- Leukaemias
- Leukaemoid reaction
- Inflammatory disorders
- Collagen disorders.

Leucopenia

A. *Physiological* Exposure to extreme cold

B. *Pathological* Infections—*Typhoid, paratyphoid, viral infection (infectious hepatitis).*
Overwhelming sepsis
Aplastic anaemia
Cytotoxic therapy
Drugs
– Chloramphenicol
– Sulpha drugs
– Aspirin
Starvation and Malnutrition
Hypersplenism.

* Values from reference no. 3

QUESTIONS

1. What are the different uses of the haemocytometer?
2. Enumerate the differences between RBC and WBC pipette.
3. Define leukaemia. How will you differentiate between leukaemia, leucocytosis and leukaemoid reaction?
4. Mention the causes of leucocytosis.
5. Name one condition where WBC pipette is used for RBC count and vice versa.

EXPERIMENT NO. 8

AIM: TOTAL RED BLOOD CELL COUNT

Principle

As the RBC count is in millions, it can be made possible only by counting RBCs in a known volume of blood by diluting with known amount of diluting fluid. The number of RBCs in undiluted blood is calculated considering the dilution factor.

Reagents and Apparatus

1. Hayem's Fluid (RBC Diluting Fluid)

a. Sodium chloride 0.50 g: It maintains isotonicity so that RBCs remain suspended in the fluid.
b. Sodium sulphate 2.50 g: It acts as an anticoagulant and prevents rouleaux formation.
c. Mercuric chloride ($HgCl_2$) 0.25 g: It acts as a preservative, anti-fungal and anti-bacterial agent.
d. Distilled water 100 ml.

2. Other Diluting Fluids

a. Toisson's fluid
b. Formaldehyde: A solution of 10 ml of 40% formalin, made up to one litre with 32 g/L trisodium citrate. It maintains the normal disc shape of RBCs and prevents agglutination. Cells are preserved and counts can be performed several hours after dilution of blood.

3. Haemocytometer Consisting of

a. *Neubauer's* chamber: The counting chamber was originally invented by Crammer in 1885 and was later modified by *Neubauer*. It is used to obtain a very thin film of fluid of known volume for cellular counts. It consists of a thick glass slide with a polished central platform divided by a short transverse gutter into two portions, each portion of which is ruled with a counting grid. On either side, the central platform is bounded by a groove called as moat. Each moat, in turn is bounded on its outer side by another platform, which is slightly higher than the central platform. A perfectly ground cover slip rests upon the two lateral platforms, thus bridging the moats and covering the central platform. The chamber is so constructed that there is a space of 0.1 mm between the ruled platform and the cover slip. The counting grid is made up of a ruled area measuring 3 mm × 3 mm. This area is divided by triple lines into 9 large equal squares each having an area of 1 sq mm. (1 mm × 1 mm). Of these the 4 large squares at the corners are used for WBC counting while the large square in the centre is used for RBC count. The large central square is divided into 25 medium squares. Each medium square is further divided into 16 small squares.
b. Cover slip
c. RBC pipette: It is a capillary pipette which is dilated near one end into a bulb. There are three markings 0.5, 1 below the bulb and 101 above the bulb of the pipette. Bulb contains a red bead which helps in mixing of blood with diluting fluid and helps in differentiating RBC pipette with WBC pipette.

4. Sterile Pricking Needle, Cotton, Spirit

5. Microscope

Procedure

- The finger is pricked under aseptic conditions
- The first drop of blood is discarded. The pipette is held in horizontal position and the blood is drawn up to mark 0.5 and the extra blood adhering to the tip of the pipette and adjoining surface is wiped off
- Immediately the Hayem's fluid is sucked up to mark 101
- Blood and the fluid are thoroughly mixed by rotating the pipette in between the palms and one minute waiting time is given
- A cover slip is placed on the Neubauers chamber symmetrically over the ruled area
- The Neubauers chamber is focused under low power objective of the microscope and RBC counting squares are brought into focus
- The Neubauers chamber is removed without disturbing the focus of the microscope and placed on the table
- The first few drops of the pipette are to be discarded
- A small drop of fluid is allowed to be formed at the tip of the pipette and the drop is gently touched to the edge of the cover slip. The fluid is allowed to spread by capillary action between the chamber and cover slip. This is known as charging of the chamber
- If fluid over flows into the trenches, it is overcharging and if it is insufficient to fill the chamber it is called undercharging. If it is over or under charged the process is repeated
- The chamber is placed under low power objective of the microscope already brought to the focus
- Finally the cells are focused under high power objective using fine adjustment
- After making sure that the cells are uniformly distributed the count is performed over the large central square meant for RBC count. The large central square (1 mm × 1 mm) is divided into 25 medium squares. Each medium square is further divided into 16 smaller squares. RBCs are counted in four corners medium squares and one central square of the large central counting area.

Rules for Counting

In order to avoid repetitive counting of cells lying on the borders, (with half of the cells projecting in one small square and half in another small square), cells lying on the left and upper border are omitted while those lying on right and lower border are counted and vice versa.

Calculation

1. *Dilution factor*

   As the initial '1' part of the pipette does not contain blood, this is deducted from '101'. Hence, 0.5 parts of blood are diluted in 100

   Therefore, 1 part is diluted in 200 and the dilution factor is 1 in 200
2. *Volume of the diluted blood in 5 medium RBC squares*

   Area of one medium square = $\frac{1}{5}\text{mm} \times \frac{1}{5}\text{mm} = \frac{1}{25}\text{mm}^2$

Area of one medium square = $5 \times \frac{1}{25} mm = \frac{1}{5} mm^2$

Depth of each chamber = 0.1 mm

Therefore, volume of 5 RBC squares = $1/5\ mm^2 \times 1/10$ mm

= $1/50\ mm^3$

3. *Total RBC count*

The number of cells counted in $1/50\ mm^3$ of diluted blood = N

Therefore, number of cells in 1 mm^3 of undiluted blood will be = N × 50 × 200 (dilution factor)

= N × 10,000 million RBC/mm^3

Normal Values

- 5–6.5 million/mm^3 in males
- 4–5.5 million/mm^3 in females.

Precautions

- The finger should not be squeezed to form a blood drop as tissue fluid might dilute the blood and this lowers the RBC count
- Pipette should be dry
- Neubauer chamber and cover slip should be cleaned properly
- Cover slip should be symmetrically placed
- Fluid in the stem of the pipette should be discarded up to mark '1'
- There should be no under or over charging of the chamber and cells are allowed to settle down.
- The cells should be uniformly distributed
- Rules for the counting of the cells should be followed so as to avoid recounting of the same cell
- RBCs should be differentiated from the dust particles as RBCs have regular size and shape and are bright round bodies while dust particles are of irregular size and shape and disappear with change of focus.

Differences between RBC and WBC Pipette

1. RBC pipette has three markings 0.5, 1 and 101 whereas WBC pipette has markings as 0.5, 1 and 11, as dilution is 200 and 20 respectively.
2. The bulb of RBC pipette is larger than that of the WBC pipette.
3. RBC pipette contains red glass bead while WBC pipette contains white glass bead.

Other Uses of RBC Pipette

1. WBC counting in leukaemia
2. Sperm counting
3. Platelet counting.

QUESTIONS

1. Mention the units of marking on the RBC pipette and mention the dilution factor.
2. Enumerate the sources of error in RBC count by manual method. Name any other accurate method for determination of RBC count.
3. Mention the alternate fluids used for RBC count.

EXPERIMENT NO. 9

AIM: DETERMINATION OF BLOOD GROUPS

Principle

The red cells bear different antigens on their membrane surface, which are glycoproteins. These are known as agglutinogens. Blood group antigens of different systems are glycolipids, oligosaccharides etc. Plasma contains antibodies or agglutinins. The red cell antigens are allowed to react with sera containing known antibodies, which results in agglutination that is detected by naked eye as well as under the microscope indicating blood group of the individual.

Apparatus and Reagents

1. Microscope
2. Sterile finger pricking needle/lancet
3. Cotton
4. Spirit
5. Glass slides
6. Stirrer
7. Glass marking pencils
8. Glass dropper
9. Normal saline.

Antisera

Antiserum A (containing α agglutinin derived from B blood group donor).
Antiserum B (containing β agglutinin derived from A blood group donor).
Antiserum D (containing D agglutinin).

Procedure

- Glass slides are cleaned and marked with a glass marking pencil
- One slide is divided into 2 parts by marking with pencil as part A and part B
- Two other slides are marked as D and S
- Six to eight drops of normal saline are placed in the middle of the slide marked S
- Finger is pricked using aseptic precautions and 2 big drops of blood are added to the saline on the slide S and mixed well to make red cell suspension
- One drop of antiserum A is placed on the part of the slide marked A and one drop of antiserum B is placed on the part marked B
- A drop of antiserum D is placed on the slide marked D
- One drop of red cell suspension is added to each of the antisera and mixed well by using separate glass rods or stirrer
- After 12–15 minutes, the slides are examined with naked eye as well as under microscope after placing cover slip, for any agglutination
- Red cell suspension on slide S is taken as control.

Haemolysis

It is rupture of RBCs (laking of blood) and this destroys RBC membrane and hence should be avoided before performing a test.

Agglutination

It is due to the antigen-antibody interaction where the molecules come close by cross linking to produce visible clumping.

Interpretation of Results

Agglutination of RBCs appears as a coarse separation of red cells into dark red clumps and brick red tinging of the serum while if RBCs form rouleaux the sedimented cells show orange tint of the red cell suspension. Presence or absence of agglutination of the red cells indicates blood group of the individual.

Antiserum A (α agglutinin)	*Antiserubm B (β agglutinin)*	*Agglutinogen on RBCs*	*Agglutinin in plasma*	*Blood group*
+	–	A	β	A
–	+	B	α	B
+	+	AB	Nil	AB
–	–	Nil	α, β	O
+ agglutination; – No agglutination				

Rh (D) Blood Grouping

Antiserum D (D agglutinin)	*Agglutinogen*	*Blood Group*
Agglutination +	RBC contain Rh (D) antigen	Rh+ve
Agglutination –	Rh (D) is absent on RBC	Rh-ve

1. False positive results are due to rouleaux formation, which should be excluded by comparing with control (red cell suspension acts as control).
2. False negative results are due to decreased *immunocompetency of antisera* (because of prolonged and improper storage or expiry of antisera).
3. Clot formation, haemolysis should be excluded.

Precautions

- Slide should be clean and dry to avoid haemolysis and marked properly
- The blood should not form a clot before mixing with saline
- While Red cell suspension is being mixed thoroughly with antisera, care must be taken not to mix two sera (Anti A and Anti B) on same glass slide
- If there is no clumping, wait for 15 minutes
- Diluted blood is used as undiluted blood may give false positive result due to rouleaux formation
- It should be examined before the preparation dries up
- Agglutination should not be confused with clot formation
- Agglutination should be confirmed microscopically.

Clinical Significance

- To ensure compatible blood transfusion
- To prevent the *haemolytic disease of newborn*
- Paternity dispute/settlement
- Medico-legal problems.

Cross Matching

It is a pre transfusion selection procedure and has to be performed as a mandatory procedure in order to avoid haemolytic (transfusion) reactions. Blood grouping and cross matching should always be done before transfusion to ensure a safe and compatible blood transfusion and avoid early, intermediate and late reactions.

- *Major cross matching*
  In major cross matching, the cells of the donor are directly matched against the plasma of the recipient. It is important to ensure that antibodies present in the recipient's plasma do not harm the donor's red cells.
- *Minor cross matching*
  In minor cross matching the donor's plasma is checked against red cells of the recipient. It is not so important as the small volume of donor plasma is diluted in a large volume of recipient's plasma. Therefore, the titre of antibodies present in the donor's plasma falls to such a low level after transfusion that they are quite unlikely to damage the red cells of the recipient.

QUESTIONS

1. Define universal donor and universal recipient.
2. Elaborate the clinical and medico-legal significance of blood grouping.

EXPERIMENT NO. 10

AIM: TO DETERMINE BLEEDING TIME AND CLOTTING TIME

Bleeding Time (Duke's Method)

Principle

The duration from the time the deep prick is given to the cessation of the bleeding is known as bleeding time. The bleeding time depends on the function of the platelets and integrity of capillaries.

Setup

1. Sterile finger pricking lancet
2. Spirit
3. Filter/blotting paper
4. Stop watch.

Procedure

- Finger tip is cleaned with spirit and the skin is allowed to dry completely
- A deep prick is given in the finger tip and blood is allowed to flow freely (finger should not be squeezed)
- Stop watch is brought into action immediately at the time of the prick
- The drop of the blood appearing on the finger tip is blotted/absorbed by using the filter paper or blotting paper at every 15 seconds (do not allow the filter paper to press on the bleeding spot).

Observation

The drop of the blood becomes smaller progressively. The time of stoppage of bleeding is noted. Number of drops of blood on filter paper are to be counted and multiplied by 15 seconds and the result is expressed in minutes and fraction of minutes.

Note: If bleeding does not stop in 10 minutes pressure is applied to the bleeding spot to stop bleeding.

Normal Value

Bleeding time is 1–5 minutes.

Precautions

- Aseptic procedures are to be followed
- Do not rub while cleaning the skin as rubbing increases the blood flow and alters the bleeding time
- Puncture should be deep enough and blood should flow freely (don't squeeze)
- Time of blotting the drop should be exactly once every 15 seconds
- Do not press on the bleeding spot as it may interfere with bleeding and alters bleeding time
- If blood continues after 10 minutes, apply pressure on the spot so as to arrest bleeding.

Clinical Significance

Causes of Prolongation of Bleeding Time

1. *Thrombocytopenia*
   - Due to decreased production of platelets
     a. *Aplastic anaemia*
     b. *Leukaemia, disseminated cancers (due to marrow infiltration)*
     c. *Drugs, e.g. alcohol, cytotoxic drugs, thiazides.*
     d. *Infections, e.g. Human immunodeficiency virus (HIV), measles*
     e. *Megaloblastic anaemia (folic acid and vitamin B_{12} deficiency)*
   - Due to increased destruction of platelets
     a. *Immunological destruction (idiopathic thrombocytopenic purpura)*
        - Post transfusion and neonatal thrombocytopenia
        - Drugs e.g. heparin, sulpha drugs
        - Infections e.g. Human immunodeficiency virus, Cytomegalovirus
     b. *Non-immunological destruction*
        - Disseminated intravascular coagulation
        - Thrombotic thrombocytopenic purpura
        - Microangiopathic haemolytic anaemia (due to mechanical injury)
     c. *Hypersplenism* (Increased sequestration of platelets)
     d. *Transfusion of blood stored for more than 24 hours in large amounts*
2. *Defects in function of platelets*
   - Haemolytic thrombasthenia
   - vonWillebrands disease
   - Drugs e.g, aspirin, large doses of penicillin
   - Uraemia
   - Leukaemia
   - Cirrhosis
3. *Vessel wall defects*
   - Prolonged treatment with drugs—Aspirin, corticosteroids, penicillin, sulpha drugs
   - Allergic purpura
   - Infections—Haemolytic streptococci, *Typhus, bacterial endocarditis*
   - Deficiency of vitamin C
   - Senile purpura—Due to loss of elastic and connective tissues around vessels.

Other Methods

Bleeding time by Ivy method: A sphygmomanometer is applied on the upper arm and blood pressure is raised to 40 mm of Hg and maintained. An incision is made on the forearm 5 cm below the cubital fossa on the anterior aspect. The length of the time is noted for cessation of bleeding. Normal bleeding time by this method is 5-11 minutes at 37°C. It is more reliable than Duke's method but is painful to the subject.

Clotting Time (Capillary Glass Tube Method)

Principle

Blood from fingertip is taken into a capillary glass tube and the length of time starting from finger prick to the formation of a thin strand of fibrin, known as clotting time is noted.

Apparatus

1. Sterile lancet/needle
2. Capillary tube (10–15 cm long and 1 mm in diameter)
3. Spirit
4. Cotton swab
5. Stop watch.

Procedure

- Procedure is to be explained to the subject
- Finger is pricked by sterile lancet and blood is allowed to flow freely
- Stop watch is started immediately at the time of prick
- A large drop of blood is obtained and is allowed to fill the capillary tube by dipping its one end into the drop by capillary action
- The capillary is placed in between palms to maintain the body temperature
- At the end of one minute, 1 cm of the capillary is broken off. This procedure is to be repeated at every 30 seconds till there is appearance of a thin thread/strand of fibrin in between two broken ends of the tube
- Stop watch is stopped immediately and time is noted.

Normal Value of Clotting Time is 2–8 Minutes

Clinical Significance

Clotting time is prolonged in the following conditions:

1. *Hereditary Causes*
   i. Clotting factor deficiencies
      – *Haemophilia A*
      – *Haemophilia B*
      – *Afibrinogenaemia*
      – *Deficiency of factor XIII*
   ii. von Willebrands disease
2. *Acquired Causes*
   i. Vitamin K deficiency and disorders of fat absorption
   ii. Liver disease
   iii. Anticoagulant therapy
   iv. Disseminated intravascular coagulation
   v. Massive transfusion of stored blood (V and VIII deficiency)
   vi. Circulating inhibitors of coagulation.

Other Methods

1. *Lee and white test tube method:* It is more reliable and sensitive method. Venous blood is collected in glass tube at 37°C. Time taken by the blood to clot is noted and this is the clotting time. Normal clotting time is 5–12 minutes by this method.
2. *Dropmethod:* Itislessaccurate. Adropofbloodisplacedonaglassslideandapinisdippedintoblooddropevery 30 seconds and time is noted when fibrin thread adheres to the pin.

Other Methods Employed for Disorders of Haemostasis

a. Clot retraction time: Blood is collected in a glass tube/vial without an anticoagulant. The clot of blood begins to shrink/retract in 30 minutes and leaves a straw coloured fluid, i.e. serum. It is 50% within one hour and completes in 24 hrs. Clot retraction depends on factors released by platelets.
b. Platelet count
c. Capillary fragility test
d. Clot lysis time
e. Prothrombin time
f. Thrombin time
g. Platelet aggregation test
h. Platelet adhesiveness test.

QUESTIONS

1. Mention the clinical significance of bleeding time and clotting time.
2. Why is the clotting time more than bleeding time?
3. Comment on different methods for determining bleeding time and clotting time.

EXPERIMENT NO. 11

AIM: DETERMINATION OF ABSOLUTE VALUES

Principle

Absolute values are derived from RBC count, haemoglobin concentration and Packed Cell Volume and are widely used in the classification of the anaemias.

Following are the absolute values:
1. MCV—Mean Corpuscular Volume
2. MCH—Mean Corpuscular Haemoglobin
3. MCHC—Mean Corpuscular Haemoglobin Concentration
4. Colour index.

Procedure

Haemoglobin concentration, total RBC count and packed cell volume are determined.
Calculations

A. *MCV (Mean Corpuscular Volume):* It is the average volume of the red blood cells expressed in cubic microns.

$$\text{MCV} = \frac{\text{PCV in \%}}{\text{RBC count in millions/mm}^3} \times 10\ \mu\text{m}^3$$

Multiplication factor 10 is for conversion of PCV (in percentage) from volume of packed red cells per 100 ml to volume per litre.
Normal Values

Adults	74–94 μm^3
Newborn	106 μm^3
Infants	70–86 μm^3

B. *MCH (Mean Corpuscular Haemoglobin)*

It is the average haemoglobin content of a red cell expressed in picograms.

$$\text{MCH} = \frac{\text{Hb (gm/dl)}}{\text{RBC count in millions/mm}^3} \times 10 \text{ picograms}$$

Normal Values
27–32 picograms.

C. *MCHC (Mean Corpuscular Haemoglobin Concentration)*

It is the average haemoglobin concentration per unit volume of the packed red cells. It is expressed as percentage:

$$\text{MCHC} = \frac{\text{Hb (gm/dl)}}{\text{PCV (\%)}} \times 100\%$$

Normal Values
31–35%.

Clinical Significance

1. MCV
   If it is less than 70 μm^3, it indicates microcytosis and elevated MCV more than 96 μm^3 indicates macrocytosis.
   Causes of Microcytosis
   - Iron deficiency anaemia
   - Thalassaemia.

   Causes of Macrocytosis
   Megaloblastic anaemia due to Vitamin B_{12} or folic acid deficiency.
   Significant rise in the number of reticulocytes which are larger than RBC also produce macrocytosis.
2. MCH
   It may be as high as 50 picogram in macrocytic anaemia or as low as 20 picograms or less in hypochromic microcytic anaemia.
3. MCHC
   It is a more reliable index as it expresses the haemoglobin concentration in relation to cell volume rather than RBC count. Decreased MCHC indicates interference with synthesis of haemoglobin, e.g. iron deficiency anaemia, thalassaemia.
4. Colour index

It is the ratio of percentage of haemoglobin to RBC percentage. It indicates haemoglobin content of RBCs.

$$\text{Colour index} = \frac{\text{Hb percentage}}{\text{RBC percentage}} = \frac{100}{100} = 1 \text{ is the normal value}$$

Where, 14.5 g% of haemoglobin is taken as 100%
5 million/mm^3 RBC count is taken as 100%
Normal value: 0.85–1.15
Colour index is low in iron deficiency anaemia and high in macrocytic anaemia.

QUESTIONS

1. Why one can never be hyperchromic?
2. Which absolute blood index is more reliable and why?
3. Mention the clinical significance of absolute blood indices.

DEMONSTRATION NO. 1

AIM: DETERMINATION OF ERYTHROCYTE SEDIMENTATION RATE

Principle

When anticoagulated blood is allowed to stand, the red blood cells settle down due to rouleaux formation towards the bottom as the red cells are more dense than plasma. The rate at which red cells settle down in an hour is known as Erythrocyte Sedimentation Rate.

There are two methods to determine ESR:

Westergren Method

Apparatus and Reagents

1. Westergren pipette:
   It is a 30 cm long, open ended tube with internal bore diameter of 2.5 mm. It is graduated from 0-200 mm.
2. Westergren stand or rack:
   It is to accommodate westergren tube in vertical position and provided with rubber pads at the lower end and metal clips at the upper end. It can accommodate six tubes at a time.
3. Disposable syringe and needle (2 ml).
4. Spirit and cotton swab.
5. 3.8% sodium citrate.
   It acts as an anticoagulant, 4 parts of blood are mixed with 1 part of sodium citrate.

Procedure

- Venous blood (1.6 ml) is withdrawn from antecubital vein. This is diluted with 0.4 ml of anticoagulant. This gives 1:4 ratio of anticoagulant to blood
- Westergren pipette is filled slowly with anticoagulant mixed blood exactly up to mark zero, keeping the finger at the upper end of the tube (it should not have any air bubbles)
- Pipette is transferred vertically to the stand by firmly pressing its lower end to the rubber pads so as to avoid leakage of the blood and screw cap is tied
- Reading should be taken at the end of 1 hour and 2 hours.

Normal Values

Male : 0–8 mm in 1st hr
Females : 8–16 mm in 1st hr

Precautions

- Proper amount of anticoagulant should be used
- As temperature affects ESR, it should be done at room temperature. High temperature and low temperature give false high and low values respectively
- Tube should be vertically placed as tilting will increase ESR
- Time should be accurate as the rate of sedimentation is slow in beginning and fast after 45 minutes
- Subject should be in fasting state.

Wintrobe's Method

Apparatus and Reagents

1. Wintrobe's tube
   It is a 12 cm long tube with bore diameter of 2 mm. It is graduated from 0–100 mm from above downwards for ESR and 0–100 mm from below upwards for haematocrit.
2. Wintrobe's rack or stand
   It is a wooden rack with holes for holding wintrobe's tube.
3. Disposable syringe and needle (2 ml)
4. Spirit swab
5. Pasteur pipette:
   It has a long thin nozzle with neck and bulb.
6. Blood sample:
   Double oxalate or fresh EDTA is used as an anticoagulant.

Procedure

- Using aseptic precautions, 2 ml of blood is withdrawn from antecubital vein and emptied into a vial containing double oxalate and mixed well
- Wintrobe's tube is filled up to mark 0 with pasteur pipette
- Tip of the pipette should be introduced right down to the bottom of the Wintrobe's tube and blood is slowly poured out of the pipette into the tube. This will prevent formation of air bubbles
- Wintrobe's tube is then placed in vertical position in the stand and allowed to stand undisturbed for 1 hour
- Reading is taken after 1 hour.

Normal Values

Male 4–10 mm in Ist hr
Female 6–12 mm in Ist hr

Precautions

- Wintrobe's tube and pipette should be clean
- Blood should be mixed with anticoagulant thoroughly
- Blood should be filled exactly up to '0' mark
- There should be no air bubbles in the tube and tube should be kept vertical as tilting will increase ESR
- Timing should be accurate
- Experiment should be done at room temperature as it varies the values of ESR.

Clinical Significance

Causes of Increased ESR

1. *Physiological* After food intake
   Pregnancy (due to increased fibrinogen and haemodilution)
   Menstruation

	Exercise (due to increased body temperature)
	Old age—plasma viscosity is less
	Females—as RBC count is low.
2. *Pathological*	Acute and chronic infections
	Anaemia of all types
	Collagen disorders
	Malignancy
	Paraprotein producing disorders such as *macroglobulinaemia.*

Causes of Decreased ESR

1. *Physiological*	Infants (due to Polycythaemia)
	High altitude.
2. *Pathological*	Polycythaemia
	Afibrinogenaemia
	Sickle cell anaemia
	Hereditary spherocytosis.

QUESTIONS

1. Enumerate the factors that influence the erythrocyte sedimentation rate.
2. Why the erythrocyte sedimentation rate is more in females?

DEMONSTRATION NO. 2

AIM: TO DETERMINE THE PACKED CELL VOLUME

Principle

Anticoagulant is added to a sample of blood and centrifuged in a haematocrit tube. Red blood cells and other cellular elements of blood being heavier than plasma get packed towards the bottom of the tube by the centrifugal force and the plasma is separated. The reading of the percentage of the blood that is made up of red blood cells is noted.

Apparatus and Reagents

1. Wintrobe's tube
2. Centrifuge machine
   It should be able to produce centrifugal force of 2300 g. The centrifuge should be standardized for speed and time by taking a reference sample and obtaining a reference value.
3. Pasteur pipette
4. Syringe and needle
5. Spirit swab
6. Blood sample to which double oxalate has been added.

Procedure

- Blood sample is collected (2 ml) using aseptic precautions and transferred to a vial having anticoagulant (double oxalate) and mixed well
- Wintrobe's tube is filled with blood exactly up to mark 10 by pasteur pipette
- To avoid air bubbles and damage to red cells, Wintrobe's tube is filled with special care. It is filled by placing the tip of the pipette at the bottom of Wintrobe's tube and filled from the bottom gradually withdrawing the pipette upwards, keeping the tip under rising column of the blood
- Wintrobe's tube is placed in one of the cups of the centrifuge and centrifugation of the sample is done first at the slow speed and then gradually by increasing to a final speed of 3000 rpm for 25 minutes
- Upper level of red cell sediment is noted. Sample is again centrifuged at 3000 rpm for 5 minutes and reading is noted and three identical consecutive readings are to be taken at 5 minutes interval
- Blood separates into 3 layers:
  a. Bottom layer of red cells with its upper level distinctly visible
  b. Middle grey white layer of WBCs and platelets called buffy layer
  c. Top layer of the plasma.

Observations

The percentage of height of red cells constitutes the haematocrit value.

$$PCV \text{ or } Haematocrit = \frac{\text{Height of packed red cells (mm)} \times 100}{\text{Height of packed red cells and plasma}}$$

Precautions

- PCV should be determined within 6 hours of collection of the blood
- Haemolysed blood should not be used (It will give low values)
- Mix the blood thoroughly with anticoagulant with its proper concentration
- Extra amount of blood in the tube is removed by dropper and not by cotton as it sucks fluid part of the blood
- There should be no air bubbles in the tube
- Blood should be centrifuged for adequate time and speed.

Microhaematocrit Method

Heparinized glass capillary tubes are filled with fresh flowing capillary blood from the finger prick and centrifuged at 12000 rpm for 3 minutes. Reading is taken from a special haematocrit reader. It is accurate and requires less quantities of blood and takes less time.

Normal Values*

Male	47 + 7%
Female	42 + 5%
Full term baby/newborn	54 + 10%
Infants	38 + 6%
Children	41 + 4%

QUESTION

1. Mention the clinical significance of packed cell volume.

* Values from reference no. 3

DEMONSTRATION NO. 3

AIM: TO DETERMINE OSMOTIC FRAGILITY OF RED BLOOD CELLS

Principle

When red blood cells are suspended in normal saline (0.9% NaCl), there is no change in their size or shape. However, when red blood cells are placed in decreasing strengths of saline, they take up the water and swell until a critical volume is reached following which they get ruptured. This is known as haemolysis. The ease with which the RBCs are broken down in hypotonic solution is called osmotic fragility of RBCs. It is expressed in terms of concentration of hypotonic solution in which the cells are haemolysed.

Apparatus and Reagents

1. Twelve glass test tubes
2. Test tube rack (metal/wooden)
3. Glass marking pencils
4. Measuring pipette (10 ml)
5. Syringe with needle (2 ml)
6. Cotton
7. Spirit and 100 ml of 1% of NaCl
8. Distilled water
9. Freshly drawn heparinized venous blood sample.

Procedure

- Test tubes are to be arranged in the rack and marked 1–12
- Using measuring pipette, required amounts of 1% NaCl and distilled water are to be added and mixed in the tubes to prepare solutions of decreasing strengths of saline
- The Ist tube contains isotonic normal saline (0.9%) and last tube has distilled water with zero tonicity
- To each tube one drop of blood is added and mixed thoroughly i.e. by gently inverting the tube once
- Test tubes are to be observed after 1 hr for the extent of haemolysis against a white background
- The tubes are centrifuged and the extent of pellet is observed.

	Test Tube No.											
Reagent	**1**	**2**	**3**	**4**	**5**	**6**	**7**	**8**	**9**	**10**	**11**	**12**
1% NaCl	4.5	4.0	3.5	3.0	2.75	2.5	2.25	2.0	1.75	1.5	1.0	0.0
Distilled water (ml)	0.5	1.0	1.5	2.0	2.25	2.5	2.75	3.0	3.25	3.5	4.0	5.0
Tonicity (Strength of NaCl (in %)	0.9	0.8	0.7	0.6	0.55	0.5	0.45	0.40	0.35	0.3	0.2	0.0

Observations

All the twelve tubes are observed for the degree of haemolysis and extent of pellet formation and the result is expressed in the range from beginning of the haemolysis to the completion of haemolysis. In the first

tube, as there is no haemolysis the pellet will be large and in the last tube, as the haemolysis is complete there is no pellet formation. Accordingly the pellet size decreases from second tube onwards.

- *Partial haemolysis*

  Supernatant fluid is pink in colour which is proportional to the degree of haemolysis i.e. colour of the supernatant fluid is increasing in depth with decreasing tonicity due to increasing haemolysis. Unruptured red cells sediment at the bottom of the tube.
- *Complete haemolysis*

  Fluid in the tube will be clear and uniformly pink without red blood cells at the bottom.
- *No haemolysis*

  A tube with no haemolysis gives a clear supernatant fluid with red cells settled at the bottom.

Precautions

- Same dropper should be used for saline and distilled water
- Test tubes should be examined exactly after 1 hour
- Haemolysis should be checked against white background
- Tube should not be disturbed while taking reading.

Normal Values

Osmotic fragility starts at 0.45 to 0.50 g/dL or % and is complete at 0.34 g/dL or %.

Clinical Significance

Decreased Osmotic Fragility

- Iron deficiency anaemia
- Sickle cell anaemia
- Thalassaemia
- After splenectomy.

Increased Osmotic Fragility

- Hereditary spherocytosis
- Congenital haemolytic anaemia.

QUESTIONS

1. Define the terms isotonic and iso-osmotic.
2. Enumerate the causes of increased osmotic fragility.

DEMONSTRATION NO. 4

AIM: TO PERFORM PLATELET COUNT (FIG. 8, PLATE 4)

Direct Method

Principle

Fresh blood is diluted with Reese-Ecker fluid, which stains the platelets and prevents coagulation of blood. Platelets are counted in Neubauer chamber and result is expressed as cells per mm^3.

Apparatus and Reagents

1. Reese-Ecker fluid—It contains:
   a. Brilliant cresyl blue 0.05 g. It stains platelets.
   b. Sodium citrate 3.80 g. It prevents coagulation, preserves RBC and makes the dye solution isotonic with blood.
   c. Formaldehyde 0.2 ml. It acts as fixative and prevents fungal growth.
   d. Distilled water 100 ml. It acts as a solvent.
2. Microscope
3. Haemocytometer (RBC pipette and Neubauer counting chamber)
4. Finger pricking needle
5. Cotton
6. Spirit
7. Cover slip.

Procedure

- RBC pipette is filled with Reese-Ecker fluid up to mark '0.5' (It prevents the clumping and disintegration of platelets which occurs if blood is taken first into the pipette)
- Finger is pricked under aseptic precautions and blood is drawn up to mark '1'. Extra blood adhering to the sides of the pipette is wiped off
- The Reese-Ecker fluid is drawn up to mark '101'. Blood and the fluid in the bulb are mixed well by rotating pipette between the palms, keeping pipette horizontally. This gives dilution of 1 into 200
- First few drops are discarded and counting chamber is charged as done for RBCs and platelets are counted in 5 RBC squares.

Calculations

Dilution factor is 1:200

Area of 1 medium square = $\frac{1}{5}\times\frac{1}{5}=\frac{1}{25}\text{ mm}^2$

Area of 5 medium squares = $5\times\frac{1}{25}=\frac{1}{5}\text{ mm}^2$

Hence, volume of 5 medium squares = $1/5 \times 1/10 = 1/50$ mm^3
Platelets counted in 1/50 mm^3 of diluted blood = N
Hence, platelets counted in 1 mm^3 of undiluted blood = N × 50 × 200/mm^3.

Indirect Method

Principle

In this method a blood film is prepared and stained with Leishman's stain and platelets are counted in relation to RBCs.

Apparatus and Reagents

1. Microscope
2. Glass slides
3. Leishman's stain
4. 14% Magnesium sulphate
5. Finger pricking lancet
6. Spirit
7. Cotton.

Procedure

- A drop of 14% magnesium sulphate solution is placed on the tip of the finger
- Finger is pricked through the drop of magnesium sulphate (it is to prevent clumping and disintegration of platelets)
- A smear is made with the diluted blood and stained with Leishman's stain
- Under oil immersion objective, platelets and red blood cells are counted
- The platelets are counted in relation to 1000 RBCs
- The normal ratio of platelets to red blood cells is determined
- Total RBC count is estimated and indirect absolute count of platelets is derived
- Normal platelet to RBC ratio is 1:20.

Calculations

If RBC count is 5 million/mm^3 and platelet ratio is 1:20 then indirect absolute count of platelets will be 2,50,000/mm^3 of blood.

Normal Values

Total platelet count is 2.5–5 lacs/mm^3 of blood.

Clinical Significance

Thrombocytosis—increase in platelet count.

1. Polycythemia vera
2. Primary thrombocytosis *(Myeloproliferative diseases)*
3. Chronic myeloid leukaemia
4. Iron deficiency anaemia

5. Chronic infections
6. Surgery
7. Haemorrhage
8. Splenectomy.

Thrombocytopenia—decrease in platelet count.

1. Decreased production
   a. Bone marrow suppression due to drugs like chloramphenicol, sulpha drugs and due to radiation
   b. Aplastic anaemia
   c. Bone marrow invasion by leukemic cells and malignant cells
   d. Acute septic fevers.
2. Decreased survival and increased destruction:
   a. Idiopathic thrombocytopenic purpura
   b. Drugs—Thiazides, Quinidine, Penicillin etc.
   c. Sequestration in spleen
   d. Disseminated intravascular coagulation
   e. Haemorrhage, extensive transfusion.

QUESTION

1. Mention the clinical significance of determining platelet count.

DEMONSTRATION NO. 5

AIM: TO PERFORM TOTAL RETICULOCYTE COUNT (FIG. 9, PLATE 4)

Principle

The nuclei of red cells are lost during development. However, the cytoplasmic RNA content remains as a network in reticulocytes, which can be detected by staining the cells with supravital stains.

Supravital Stains

These are the stains which contain dyes that are used for staining the living cells.

Reticulocyte Stain

- It is a type of supravital stain consisting of:
  - Brilliant cresyl blue dye 1 g
  - 100 ml of citrated saline (1 volume of 3.8% sodium citrate and 4 volumes of sodium chloride)
- Brilliant cresyl blue: It stains RNA of reticulocyte
- Sodium citrate: It prevents coagulation
- Sodium chloride: It provides isotonicity.

Apparatus and Reagents

1. Microscope, glass slides
2. Sterile pricking needle
3. Cotton swab
4. Spirit
5. Leishman's stain
6. Reticulocyte stain.

Procedure

- Glass slide is cleaned properly
- A drop of reticulocyte stain is placed on glass slide at one end
- Finger is pricked using aseptic precautions
- An equal sized drop of blood is added to the stain and mixed with the help of a pin and allowed to remain for 1 minute
- A thin smear is made and dried and then counter stained with Leishman's stain
- Smear is first examined under low power for uniformity of distribution of red cells and then focused under oil immersion
- Reticulocytes have fine, deep violet filaments arranged in a network
- For counting, an area of the film is chosen where the cells are undistorted and the staining is good
- The RBCs and reticulocytes are enumerated by counting 1000 cells.

Calculations

$$\text{Percentage of reticulocytes} = \frac{\text{Total No. of reticulocytes counted}}{\text{Total No. of RBCs and reticulocytes}} \times 100$$

Normal Values

Adults and children : 0.2–2.0%
Infants : 2–6%

Reticulocytosis

1. *Physiological*
   - Newborn and infants
   - High altitude
   - Moderate to severe exercise
   - Menstruation.
2. *Pathological*
   - Haemolytic anaemia
   - Acute haemorrhage
   - During the response with treatment of anaemias.

Reticulocytopenia

- Aplastic anaemia
- Myxoedema
- Hypopituitarism
- Leucoerythroblastic anaemia (Presence of immature red cells and myeloid cells due to infiltration of bone marrow by abnormal structures, e.g. secondary carcinoma of bone, *myelofibrosis, multiple myeloma* and after *splenectomy*).

QUESTION

1. Describe the reticulocyte response and mention the clinical significance of reticulocyte count.

Chapter

8 Vertical Orientation Programme

1. VISIT TO DEPARTMENT OF MEDICINE

Describe your experience and benefits derived from your visit to department of medicine to learn about echocardiography, Holter monitoring and treadmill test.

2. VISIT TO DEPARTMENT OF PULMONARY MEDICINE

Describe the experience and benefits achieved from your visit to department of pulmonary medicine to learn about various pulmonary function tests.

3. VISIT TO DEPARTMENT OF OTORHINOLARYNGOLOGY(ENT)

Describe your experience and benefits derived from your visit to department of ENT to learn about audiometry.

4. VISIT TO DIETETICS DEPARTMENT

Describe the experience and benefits achieved from your visit to dietetics department to learn about balanced diet and diet regimens in different diseased states.

5. VISIT TO DEPARTMENT OF TRANSFUSION MEDICINE

Describe your experiences and benefits derived/knowledge gained from your visit to the department of Transfusion Medicine to learn about the safe blood transfusion procedures and live demonstrations.

Bibliography

1. A Textbook of Practical Physiology by C L Ghai, Jaypee Publisher, 1999.
2. Cooper K. The Aerobics Way. New York: Bantam Books Inc. 1982.
3. De Gruchy's Clinical Haematology in Medical Practice by Frank Firkin, Colin Chesterman, David Penington and Bryan Rush, Rekha Printers Pvt. Ltd., and Neil O'Brien, Oxford University, Press, 1994.
4. Ewing DJ. Cardiovascular reflex and autonomic neuropathy. Clin Sci Molec Med 1978;55, 321–7.
5. Harrison's Principles of Internal Medicine. McGraw-Hill Publishing Div. 2001.
6. Hines EA, Brown GE. The cold pressor test for measuring the reactibility of the blood pressure: Data concerning 571 normal and hypertensive subjects. Am Heart J. 1936;11:1–9.
7. Levin AB. A simple test of cardiac function based upon the heart rate changes induced by Valsalva manoeuvre. Am J Cardiol. 1966;18:90–9.
8. Manual of Practical Physiology by AK Jain, Avichal Publishing Company, 2001.
9. Practical Haematology by Sir John V Dacie, Churchill Livingstone, 1991.
10. Robbin's Pathologic basis of Diseases by Cotran, Kumar, Robbins, Prism Books Pvt. Ltd., Indian edition, 1994.
11. Swash M. Hutchison's Clinical Methods. WB Saunders 2002.
12. Textbook of Practical Physiology by GK Pal and Pravati Pal, Oriental Longman Limited, 2001.
13. Wintrobe's Clinical Haematology by G Richard Lee, Thomas C. Bithell, John Forester, John W. Athens, John N Lukens by Williams and Wilkins, 1993.
14. www.brianmac.demon.co.uk.